HARRIET ROTH'S COMPLETE GUIDE TO FATS, CALORIES, AND CHOLESTEROL

HARRIET ROTH'S COMPLETE GUIDE TO FATS, CALORIES, AND CHOLESTEROL

by
Harriet Roth

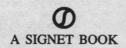

A SIGNET BOOK

SIGNET
Published by the Penguin Group
Penguin Books USA Inc., 375 Hudson Street,
New York, New York 10014, U.S.A.
Penguin Books Ltd, 27 Wrights Lane,
London W8 5TZ, England
Penguin Books Australia Ltd, Ringwood,
Victoria, Australia
Penguin Books Canada Ltd, 10 Alcorn Avenue,
Toronto, Ontario, Canada M4V 3B2
Penguin Books (N.Z.) Ltd, 182–190 Wairau Road,
Auckland 10, New Zealand

Penguin Books Ltd, Registered Offices:
Harmondsworth, Middlesex, England

Published by Signet, an imprint of Dutton Signet, a division of Penguin Books
USA Inc. Previously published by Signet in a different version under the title
Harriet Roth's Fat Counter.

First Printing, September, 1993
10 9 8 7 6 5 4 3 2

This book is dedicated
to the memory of Joe Kirshbaum,
for his encouragement and confidence.

The best thing about the future
is that it comes one day at a time.

—Abraham Lincoln

CONTENTS

CONTENTS

CONTENTS

INTRODUCTION

The most important single change that you can make in your diet is to reduce the total fat you eat. Americans have a long-standing love affair with fat, and as a result, more than one-third of the American population is overweight. In fact, according to the Surgeon General, about 34 million people need to lose 35 pounds or more for medical reasons.* C. Everett Koop, M.D., the U.S. Surgeon General in 1988, issued the first Surgeon General's Report on Nutrition and Health. He urged the public to increase its consumption of fresh fruits, vegetables, and whole grain products and to decrease the consumption of dietary fat. He observed that "your diet can influence your long-term health prospects more than any other action you may take." People are now realizing that the key to good health and weight loss is to limit fat in the diet. Some experts have gone so far as to say, "If you cut down on your fat you will lose weight. It's as simple as that." Americans are obsessed with weight-loss diets. Yet seven out of ten of those who lose weight regain it within a year or two, often because they went on fad diets that did not deal with life-style change.

> Count the fat as food so that you'll never be fooled again.

*Excess fat in the diet may contribute to heart disease; cancer of the breast, pancreas, prostate, and colon; diabetes; high blood pressure; and, of course, obesity.

INTRODUCTION

Focus on Fat, Not Calories

Most of us want to lead the good life, and the good life begins with eating healthful foods. Although some sources have advised Americans to limit their fat consumption to no more than 30% of total calories, more recent research suggests that 20% or less of our total calories should come from fat. By eating more fruits, vegetables, cereals and grain products, and limiting animal protein (no more than 4 to 5 ounces daily), we can easily limit our fat to this percentage. The gain will be in good health—the loss in weight. Here's how to determine your allowable daily fat calories:

> The approximate number of calories consumed daily × 20% (.20) = the daily calories from fat

For example: 1500 calories × .20 = 300 calories from fats. In this case, you should consume no more than 300 calories from fat each day.

The following chart lists suggested weight levels. But remember, each person's body is affected by his or her age, activity level, and other individual differences. Higher weights generally apply to men, who tend to have more muscle and bone.

U.S.F.D.A. Suggested Weight
(without clothes or shoes)

Height	19–34 years	35 years and over
5'0"	97–128	108–138
5'1"	101–132	111–143
5'2"	104–137	115–148
5'3"	107–141	119–152
5'4"	111–146	122–157
5'5"	114–150	126–162

5'6"	118–155	130–167
5'7"	121–160	134–172
5'8"	125–164	138–178
5'9"	129–169	142–183
5'10"	132–174	146–188
5'11"	136–179	151–194
6'0"	140–184	155–199
6'1"	144–189	159–205
6'2"	148–195	164–210
6'3"	152–200	168–216
6'4"	156–205	173–222

Daily Intake of Fat and Calories

To determine the daily calories you need to reach your optimum weight, multiply your desired weight by 15 calories.

Formula: Desired weight × 15 calories = daily calories needed for optimum weight.

How many grams of fat should you eat each day?

Formula: Daily calories × .20 (20%) divided by 9 (calories in one gram of fat) = total grams of fat you should consume daily.

Although the American Heart Association recommends no more than 30% of daily calories from fat, most experts today realize that 30% is too high. Remember, we are interested in prevention, not just treatment after we already have a disease. So whether you choose 10, 15, or 20% of your calories from fat as your guideline, remember less fat is better.

Daily Calorie Level	The % of total daily calories from fat in grams		
	10%	15%	20%
	The daily target in fat grams		
1200	13	20	26
1500	17	25	33
1800	20	30	40
2000	22	33	44
2200	24	37	49
2500	28	42	56
3000	33	50	67

All Calories Are Not Created Equal

There are nine calories in every gram of fat, twice as many as in every gram of protein or carbohydrate.

Counting calories is not enough. More and more scientific evidence points to the fact that the body does not treat all calories the same. It is easier for the body to turn dietary fat into body fat than protein or carbohydrate. The body burns off 3 percent of fat calories; the rest are stored as fat in places we'd prefer they weren't. As for protein and carbohydrate metabolism, 23% of the calories are used. Carbohydrates then are not the villains in weight reduction—it's the fatty sour cream and butter you put on the baked potato and the "alfredo sauce" you put on the pasta that puts on the pounds. Here's how to calculate the number of grams of fat allowed each day to lose and then maintain your weight. Let's say you consume about 1500 calories per day.

Formula: 1500 calories × .20 (20 percent) = 300 calories from fat.

300 fat calories ÷ 9 (number of calories in a gram of fat) = 33 grams.

33 grams = the number of grams of fat allowed each day on a 1500 calorie diet.

Now, most of us have no idea of what 33 grams of fat would be. Thirty-three grams of fat is about the equivalent of 6 teaspoons of oil or 8 pats of butter! The average American consumes about 80 to 100 grams of fat per day!

Better Food Labels—At Last

Do you remember the old adage that said "It would take an act of Congress to make this change"? Well, it has finally happened. All processed foods must carry the new nutrition labels by May 1994, thanks to legislators like Senator Howard Metzenbaum, Congressman Henry Waxman, and Dr. David Kessler of the FDA.

Nutrition Facts

Serving Size ½ cup (114g)
Servings Per Container 4

Amount Per Serving

Calories 260   Calories from Fat 120

	% Daily Value*
Total Fat 13g	20%
Saturated Fat 5g	25%
Cholesterol 30 mg	10%
Sodium 660mg	28%
Total Carbohydrate 31g	11%
Dietary Fiber 0g	0%
Sugars 5g	–
Protein 5g	–

Vitamin A 4%	•	Vitamin C 2%
Calcium 15%	•	Iron 4%

* Percent Daily Values are based on a 2,000 calorie diet. Your diet values may be higher or lower depending on your calorie needs:

		Calories:	2,000	2,500
Total Fat	Less than		65g	80g
Sat. Fat	Less than		20g	25g
Cholesterol	Less than		300mg	300mg
Sodium	Less than		2,400mg	2,400mg
Total Carbohydrate			300g	375g
Fiber			25g	30g

Calories per gram:
Fat 9 • Carbohydrates 4 • Protein 4

INTRODUCTION

New Label Nutrition Facts

1. Requires more realistic servings.

2. Lists total calories plus *calories from fat* based on theory that people should get no more than 30% of calories from fat.*

3. Daily value will show how food fits into overall daily value.

4. Includes list of nutrients most important to good health based on a balanced diet of 2,000 or 2,500 caloric daily intake.

5. Lists:
   1 gram of fat = 9 calories
   1 gram of carbohydrate = 4 calories
   1 gram of protein = 4 calories

Here's how to determine the percentage of fat in a portion of food:

> Formula: Grams of fat per portion × 9 calories ÷ calories per portion × 100 = the percentage of fat

For example, one slice of mild cheddar cheese (1 ounce) has 110 calories and 9 grams of fat. Nine grams fat × nine calories = 81 grams ÷ 110 calories = 74% or (.74) fat calories. Although you have only 110 calories in a slice of this cheese, 74% of these calories come from fat and are ready to put on the pounds. Keep in mind that the most healthful range for fat is about 20% of total calories.

A good rule of thumb to follow for keeping your fat content within the healthful 20% guideline is about 2 grams of fat per 100 calories. Some foods that you eat may have more

*We, of course, recommend the more prudent 20% or less of your daily calories come from fat.

than 2 grams of fat per 100 calories while others contain less (for example, fruits, vegetables, grains, and nonfat dairy products). Obviously, an occasional high-fat "treat" is not fatal, but remember that one indulgence could be your entire fat allowance or more for the day. For example, a snack of one-half cup of oil-roasted peanuts contains 35 grams of fat, your entire fat allowance for the day on a 1500 calorie diet. Remember that the 20% fat content is only a general guideline. It's the total grams of fat consumed daily that count.

Saturated Fat—The Dangerous Culprit

We know that diets high in saturated fat contribute to heart disease by raising cholesterol levels. All saturated fat raises cholesterol. Saturated fats, which are generally solid at room temperature, are found primarily in foods of animal origin such as whole milk dairy products (butter, cream, milk, sour cream, ice cream and cheeses), and in meat, lard, chicken and beef fat. Saturated fats are also found in tropical oils such as coconut oil, palm oil, palm kernel oil, cocoa butter, and any other vegetable oil that has been hydrogenated such as stick margarine. Remember the softer the margarine, the less saturated fat it contains. (When an oil is hydrogenated, it becomes more saturated and is thus more likely to raise your cholesterol level. Tropical oils are used commercially because they are inexpensive and have a long shelf life.)

Although some food processors avoid using tropical oils (i.e., palm or coconut oil), saturated fats are still sometimes hidden in many processed foods such as bakery goods, popcorn, salad and cooking oils, bouillon cubes, crackers, and some non-dairy creamers.

I have listed the total fat grams and not listed saturated fat separately. Trying to count both saturated fat and total fat can get to be a burden that can be discouraging. Counting total fat is simple! If you limit your *total fat to below*

20% of your total calories, you will automatically be limiting your saturated fat intake.

A Few Words About Cholesterol Control

Cholesterol is a fatty, waxlike substance *that can only be found in foods of animal origin.* A food can be high in fat—like nuts, avocados or chocolate—but contain no cholesterol. That is because these foods originate from plant, not animal sources. Some foods are high in cholesterol—such as shellfish—but low in saturated fat which raises cholesterol.

I have listed the cholesterol content of foods in this book because high serum cholesterol contributes to heart disease.

> To prevent heart disease, limit your cholesterol intake to less than 100 milligrams per day.

You can do this by eating more whole grains, fruits, and vegetables, and limiting your portions of *any* animal protein to 4–5 ounces per day.

Losing Weight Is Easy—You've Done It a Hundred Times

Each year more than 50 million Americans are obsessed with going on a diet. Unfortunately, the majority regain the lost pounds, and then some. The most significant change that you can make in your life-style is to focus on the fat that you eat and count the grams of fat. By simply reducing your fat intake, weight loss will automatically follow, and you will discover that losing and maintaining weight loss is not the impossible dream.

Twelve Weight-Loss Tips

1. Count your grams of fat, not calories.

2. Keep a daily diary. Record everything that passes your lips and check to find out what, when and why you eat.

3. Keep problem foods out of the house.

4. Read food labels for fat and calories.

5. Don't skip meals. Have three meals a day and two snacks. Choose low-fat snacks such as air-popped popcorn, vegetables, fruits, non-fat yogurt, or non-fat crackers.

6. Eat more fiber and complex carbohydrates, such as salads and vegetables. Limit the added fat by asking for dressing and sauces on the side.

7. Choose "clean" food. Instead of frying—broil, bake, grill, or poach foods without fat-laden sauces.

8. Limit your animal protein to a portion the size of a deck of cards. Eat such protein no more than once a day.

9. Try to have two vegetarian days. Select from hearty soups, salads, vegetables, pastas, whole grain products, and fruit.

10. Drink an eight-ounce glass of water before each meal with a total of six to eight glasses per day.

11. Exercise regularly. Start slowly with a 15-minute walk each day and try to build to 45 minutes (about three miles), five days a week.

Exercise does not have to be aerobic in order to burn off pounds. Just walking will jump start your metabolism and speed up your weight loss. More important—it's never too late to start!

---

12. Don't give up. Choose to lose but don't get discouraged. If you goof occasionally, don't feel you've blown it—just get back on track.

INTRODUCTION

All fat can be fattening as well as unhealthful. Your goal is to reduce the overall amount of fat that you consume. How can you do this?

To Cut The Fat

1. Choose low fat foods. Stock your shelves with healthy choices.

2. Cook with little or no added fat.

3. Add as little fat as possible in sauces, salad dressings, and as a spread on bread.

4. *Limit how much you eat overall.*

Fat Facts

Do you know that:

1. All calories are not created equal. The body turns food fat into body fat more readily than protein or carbohydrates.

2. The fatter people are, the more they tend to prefer "the taste of fat."

3. Margarine has the same number of calories as butter (about 100 calories per tablespoon).

4. Americans eat 1.5 billion pounds of potato chips a year. That's an average of six pounds—and the equivalent of 870 grams of fat or about 58 tablespoons of oil—for every man, woman, and child in the country.

5. A small order of french fries contains approximately 12 grams (about 1 tablespoon) of fat.

6. Fish were not meant to swim in fat calories (i.e., butter, batter or tartar sauce).

7. A healthful salad topped with two tablespoons of regular high-fat salad dressing contains nearly as much fat as a hamburger.

8. One tablespoon of regular salad dressing contains 6 to 9 grams of fat, equivalent to two pats of margarine or butter.

9. Replacing a daily tablespoon of butter or margarine with light margarine lowers your yearly intake of calories by 18,250 or five pounds.

10. One and one-half tablespoons of half-and-half in a cup of coffee twice a day is only 40 calories a day—but one year later, you will have consumed an extra 14,600 calories and show a four-pound weight gain.

11. A doughnut is more likely to "settle on your hips" than two slices of whole wheat bread or a bagel. Calories from fatty foods are more likely to be stored as fat than those from protein or carbohydrate.

12. Lean roast beef almost always has less fat than a hamburger.

13. Extra-crispy fried chicken also contains extra fat.

14. The United States ranks number one in the percentage of adult population classified as overweight.

> Face the facts—all fat can be fattening as well as unhealthful.

15. The rarer your steak or hamburger, the more fat and calories it contains.

16. Americans spend over $50 billion a year on fast food meals.

17. The average American consumes 18 pounds of snack foods a year.

18. The softer the margarine the better; the fewer trans-fatty acids it contains. So tub or whipped margarine is

better than stick margarine; and liquid oil, whether margarine, canola or olive oil, is even better.

19. As many dietary fats fall from grace, olive oil's star continues to rise. *However, it should not be consumed with abandon.*

20. *All* oils contain 120 calories and 14 grams of fat per tablespoon.

Decisions! Decisions!

Try these lower-fat substitutions. Cut the fat, but enjoy the flavor.

	INSTEAD OF THIS	SUBSTITUTE THIS
Beverages	1 cup whole milk	1 cup skimmed milk
	1 chocolate milkshake	1 cup cocoa prepared with skimmed milk or water
	1 cup coffee with 1 tb. cream	1 cup coffee with 1% fat milk
Dressing	¼ cup sour cream	¼ cup non-fat plain yogurt
Protein	3½ oz. canned tuna in oil	3½ oz. canned tuna in water
Breakfast	3-egg cheese omelet	¾ cup Egg Beater's vegetable omelet or egg-white omelet
	Two 7-inch waffles, with butter & syrup	Four 4-inch pancakes, sugar-free jam
	Croissant & 1 cup Granola with coconut	Bagel & 1 cup whole wheat flakes

	Eggs Benedict	Poached eggs on whole wheat toast
Sandwich	Club	Turkey
	Tuna salad	Chicken breast w/o skin, grilled
	Bologna	Lean roast beef
	Grilled American cheese	Open-face light-line cheese, melted
	Cheeseburger	¼ pound plain lean hamburger or turkey burger
Soup	1 cup New England clam chowder	1 cup Manhattan clam chowder
	1 cup French onion soup with cheese	1 cup vegetarian split pea soup
	1 cup cream of tomato soup	1 cup gazpacho
	1 cup cream of chicken soup	1 cup chicken gumbo
Meat, Fish, Poultry	¼ pound regular ground sirloin	¼ pound ground turkey breast
	Porterhouse steak	4 ounce lean top sirloin
	Prime rib roast	Sirloin tip or top round roast
	3½ ounce chicken drumstick w/skin	3½ ounce chicken breast, broiled or roasted, w/o skin
	Chicken thigh	Chicken leg
	3½ ounces breaded, fried fish	1½ ounces grilled, broiled, or poached fish

	3½ ounces fried shrimp	3½ ounces boiled shrimp with cocktail sauce
	Fried crab cakes or deviled crab cakes	Steamed clams or Alaskan crab legs
	3½ ounces duck roasted, no skin	3½ ounces chicken roasted, no skin
	Rack of lamb	Leg of lamb
Fast Foods	Beef burrito	Soft chicken taco
	Double burger with cheese	¼ pound burger with bun
	Chocolate malt	Chocolate milk
	Onion rings	French fries
	Hot cakes with butter and syrup	English muffin with jam
	½ pound hamburger	Chili
	Chili without beans	Black bean chili
	Danish	Fat-free muffins
Snacks	1 ounce potato chips	1 ounce pretzels
	1 cup popcorn popped in oil	1 cup air-popped popcorn
	1 ounce chocolate	3 marshmallows
	1 ounce peanuts	2 cups air-popped popcorn
	1 Snickers bar	1 Tootsie Roll
	1 oz. Hershey's Kisses	1 oz. jelly beans
Desserts	1 slice pecan pie	1 slice apple pie (1 crust)
	Chocolate cake with icing	Angel food cake
	2 chocolate chip cookies	2 vanilla wafers

	1 cup ice cream	1 cup non-fat frozen yogurt or sorbet
Miscella-neous	1 slice pepperoni pizza	1 slice vegetarian pizza
	1 glazed doughnut	1 bagel
	1 corn muffin	1 English muffin
	1 tablespoon mayon-naise	1 tablespoon mustard
	1 ounce brown gravy	1 ounce au jus gravy
	Stick of butter or mar-garine	Light, soft margarine or olive oil
	Butter or cream cheese	Fruit spread or jam
	Cheese sauce	Tomato sauce
	Macaroni & cheese	Pasta and tomato sauce
	Regular crackers	Crispbread or flat-bread
	1 whole artichoke with hollandaise sauce	1 whole artichoke with lemon
	1 ounce cheddar cheese	1 ounce low-fat ched-dar cheese
	1 ounce Brie cheese	1 ounce low-fat goat cheese
	½ cup whole-milk cottage cheese	½ cup non-fat cottage cheese
	6 oz. baked potato with butter and sour cream	6 oz. baked potato topped with plain yogurt or non-fat sour cream
	Mashed potatoes	Boiled potato
	½ cup hash browns	½ baked potato

THE NEW FOOD PYRAMID

Government-backed nutrition advice in the 1940's was called The Basic Seven. Later it was The Four Food Groups. In the 1980's, the dietary guidelines for Americans recommended a reduction in fat and an increase in grains. In 1991, the FDA promoted a plant-based diet. They felt that one picture was worth 1,000 words, resulting in the Visual Food Guide Pyramid. It limited the amount of animal products by suggesting that you eat more food from the bottom of the pyramid than from the top. That is, eating lower on the food chain. Although the pyramid is an outline, not a definite prescription, don't forget to watch your fat consumption.

WHAT COUNTS AS A SERVING?

FOOD GROUPS

Bread, Cereal, Rice, and Pasta

1 slice of bread	1 ounce of ready-to-eat cereal	1/2 cup of cooked cereal, rice, or pasta

Vegetable

1 cup of raw leafy vegetables	1/2 cup of other vegetables, cooked, or chopped raw	3/4 cup of vegetable juice

Fruit

1 medium apple, banana, orange	1/2 cup of chopped, cooked, or canned fruit	3/4 cup of fruit juice

Milk, Yogurt, and Cheese

1 cup of milk or yogurt	1-1/2 ounces of natural cheese	2 ounces of processed cheese

**Using low-fat and non-fat dairy products
is a quick and easy way to lower your fat intake.**

Meat, Poultry, Fish, Dry Beans, Eggs, and Nuts

2-3 ounces of cooked lean meat, poultry, fish, or seafood	1/2 cup of cooked dry beans, 1 egg, or 2 tablespoons of peanut butter count as 1 ounce of lean meat

THE FOOD GUIDE PYRAMID

A Guide to Daily Food Choices

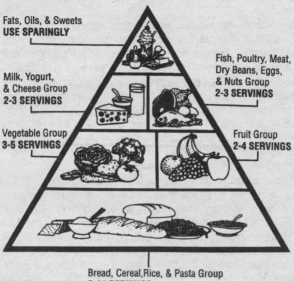

Fats, Oils, & Sweets
USE SPARINGLY

Milk, Yogurt,
& Cheese Group
2-3 SERVINGS

Fish, Poultry, Meat,
Dry Beans, Eggs,
& Nuts Group
2-3 SERVINGS

Vegetable Group
3-5 SERVINGS

Fruit Group
2-4 SERVINGS

Bread, Cereal, Rice, & Pasta Group
6-11 SERVINGS

A good diet is low in fat, cholesterol, sodium, and sugars; and high in vegetables, fruits, beans, and whole grains. Eating well can make a real difference in your health and longevity.

INTRODUCTION

The Bottom Line

Nutritionists have known for years that many over-weight people have no idea how much they eat. In fact, in recent studies the majority of people ate twice as much as they said they did. Most people are overfed and under-exercised.

Many successful recovery programs are based upon the belief of "one day at a time"—and this should be your goal in counting grams of fat. Whether it's weight reduction, disease treatment or prevention, or just wanting to feel good, this philosophy will be your greatest ally. If occasionally you indulge in that favorite dessert you lust for, or those French fries that keep calling to you, simply subtract those fat grams from another day. Don't obsess and beat yourself. Just start the next day with a positive approach to a healthful lifestyle and *choose to cut the fat*— while you are still enjoying eating.

We used to think that only calories were responsible for weight gain. We now know that the *kinds of calories we eat* are handled very differently in our bodies. Calories from fat are easier for our bodies to turn into body fat than those calories from protein or carbohydrate. A low-fat diet by itself is not a magic cure for obesity. Obviously, your genes and exercise will affect your natural body weight. However, if any style of eating is going to effectively *take off weight, keep it off*, and *keep you healthy*, you absolutely must FIGHT THE FAT.

Over 4,000 entries follow,* listing the calories, grams of fat, cholesterol, and percentage of fat, for each. It's all there for you to use. All you have to do is count the grams of fat that you eat in a day in order to keep within the healthier 20% guideline—it's as simple as that.

Some things never change, however. With the passing

---

*Recipes for all entries that are preceded by a bold asterisk can be found in *Harriet Roth's Cholesterol-Control Cookbook* (Plume, $9.95).

years, weight gain (about one pound per year after the age of 25) and concern for our health seem to increase. Choosing foods that deal with both of these concerns while still maintaining a palatable diet seems like an insurmountable obstacle. Enjoying the tastes and pleasures of good food while limiting the grams of fat is *not* the impossible dream. This book will help make your dreams a reality.

Remember—

> "Sooner or later we all sit down to a banquet of consequences."
>
> —Robert Louis Stevenson

BEVERAGES

Alcoholic

Item	PORTION	CAL-ORIES	FAT GRAMS	CHOLES-TEROL	% OF FAT
Ale, brown, bottled	12 fl. oz.	99	0.0	0	0.0
Beer					
regular	12 fl. oz.	146	0.0	0	0.0
Light, Budweiser	12 fl. oz.	110	0.0	0	0.0
Champagne	6 fl. oz.	135	0.0	0	0.0
Cider, apple, sparkling, (6.9% alcohol), Martinelli	6 fl. oz.	87	0.0	0	0.8
Coffee liqueur	1 fl. oz.	79	8.8	0	100.0
Daiquiri	6 fl. oz.	112	0.0	0	0.8
Gin					
80 proof	1½ fl. oz.	103	0.0	0	0.0
86 proof	1½ fl. oz.	111	0.0	0	0.0
90 proof	1½ fl. oz.	117	0.0	0	0.0
100 proof	1½ fl. oz.	131	0.0	0	0.0
Piña colada	6 fl. oz.	262	2.7	0	9.3
Rum					
80 proof	1½ fl. oz.	103	0.0	0	0.0
86 proof	1½ fl. oz.	111	0.0	0	0.0
90 proof	1½ fl. oz.	117	0.0	0	0.0
100 proof	1½ fl. oz.	131	0.0	0	0.0
Sherry, medium	6 fl. oz.	210	0.0	0	0.0
Tequila Sunrise	6 fl. oz.	189	0.2	0	1.0
Vodka					
80 proof	1½ fl. oz.	103	0.0	0	0.0
86 proof	1½ fl. oz.	111	0.0	0	0.0
90 proof	1½ fl. oz.	117	0.0	0	0.0
100 proof	1½ fl. oz.	131	0.0	0	0.0
Whiskey					
80 proof	1½ fl. oz.	103	0.0	0	0.0
86 proof	1½ fl. oz.	111	0.0	0	0.0
90 proof	1½ fl. oz.	117	0.0	0	0.0
100 proof	1½ fl. oz.	131	0.0	0	0.0

■ Contains less than 20% fat

Item	PORTION	CAL-ORIES	FAT GRAMS	CHOLES-TEROL	% OF FAT
Wine, dessert (18.8% alcohol)					
Dry	6 fl. oz.	224	0.0	0	0.0
Sweet	6 fl. oz.	272	0.0	0	0.8
Wine, table (12.2% alcohol)					
Muscatelle	6 fl. oz.	279	0.0	0	0.0
Red, dry	6 fl. oz.	121	0.0	0	0.0
White, dry	6 fl. oz.	124	0.0	0	0.8
White, medium dry	6 fl. oz.	133	0.0	0	0.8
Wine spritzer	6 fl. oz.	91	0.0	0	0.8
Non-Alcoholic					
■Apple-Cranberry Drink, Hi-C	6 fl. oz.	90	0.01	0	0.1
■Apple drink, Johanna Farms Ssips	8.45 fl. oz.	130	0.0	0	0.0
■Beer, non-alcoholic, Sharp's	12 fl. oz.	68	0.0	0	0.8
■Berry citrus drink, Five Alive	6 fl. oz.	88	0.01	0	0.1
■Coca-Cola	12 fl. oz.	154	0.0	0	0.0
Classic	12 fl. oz.	144	0.0	0	0.0
Dietetic	12 fl. oz.	0	0.0	0	0.0
Coconut cream, canned, sweetened	8 fl. oz.	568	52.5	0	83.2
■Coffee, regular, brewed	6 fl. oz.	4	0.0	0	0.8
Coffee, flavored, General Mills					
Cafe Amaretto	6 fl. oz.	49	2.1	0	38.6
Cafe Vienna	6 fl. oz.	60	2.1	0	31.5
Swiss Mocha	6 fl. oz.	50	3.0	0	54.0
■Coffee					
Instant	6 fl. oz.	11	0.0	0	0.8
Decaffeinated	6 fl. oz.	4	0.0	0	0.8
Prepared	6 fl. oz.	4	0.0	0	0.8
■Cranapple juice drink, Ocean Spray	6 fl. oz.	127	.01	0	0.0

Item	PORTION	CAL-ORIES	FAT GRAMS	CHOLES-TEROL	% OF FAT
■Cranberry apple drink, Town House	6 fl. oz.	130	0.0	0	0.0
■Crangrape drink, Ocean Spray	6 fl. oz.	130	0.2	0	1.4
■Dr Pepper, cola	12 fl. oz.	146	0.0	0	0.0
Eggnog (see Dairy and Dairy Products, milk)					
■Fresca	12 fl. oz.	3	0.0	0	0.0
■Fruit punch					
Canned, Hi-C	6 fl. oz.	96	0.01	0	0.1
Chilled, Minute Maid	6 fl. oz.	91	0.1	0	0.9
Mix, regular, Funny Face, prepared	6 fl. oz.	66	0.0	0	0.0
Mix, dietetic, Crystal Light	6 fl. oz.	2	0.0	0	0.0
■Gatorade, citrus flavor	1 cup	42	0.0	0	0.0
■Ginger beer	12 fl. oz.	121	0.0	0	0.0
■Grapeade, Minute Maid, chilled or frozen, prepared	6 fl. oz.	94	0.01	0	0.1
■Grape drink					
w/vitamin C	½ cup	56	0.0	0	0.8
canned, Hi-C	6 fl. oz.	96	0.1	0	1.0
Mix, prepared, Funny Face	6 fl. oz.	66	0.0	0	0.0
■Grapefruit juice cocktail, Ocean Spray	6 fl. oz.	80	0.1	0	1.1
■Juice					
Apple, canned or bottled	½ cup	58	0.1	0	1.5
Apple-cherry, canned, Red Cheek	6 fl. oz.	113	0.0	0	0.0

■ Contains less than 20% fat   3

Item	PORTION	CAL-ORIES	FAT GRAMS	CHOLES-TEROL	% OF FAT
Apple-grape, canned, Mott's	8.45 fl. oz.	128	0.0	0	0.0
Blackberry, un-sweetened, canned	½ cup	45	0.7	0	14.0
Carrot, canned	½ cup	66	0.2	0	2.7
Cranberry, Ocean Spray	6 fl. oz.	103	0.0	0	0.0
Cranberry-apple, w/vitamin C	½ cup	82	0.0	0	0.8
Grape, canned, Town House	6 fl. oz.	120	0.0	0	0.0
Grape, frozen, Ocean Spray, prepared	6 fl. oz.	200	0.0	0	0.0
Grape, sparkling, red, Welch's	6 fl. oz.	117	0.0	0	0.8
Grapefruit Canned					
Unsweetened, Ocean Spray	6 fl. oz.	70	0.2	0	2.6
Sweetened, Ardmore Farms	6 fl. oz.	78	0.2	0	2.3
Frozen, unsweet-ened, Minute Maid, prepared	6 fl. oz.	83	0.3	0	3.2
Grapefruit-orange, canned, Ardmore Farms	6 fl. oz.	78	0.2	0	2.5
Orange, fresh	½ cup	56	0.2	0	3.2
Orange Canned, Land O'Lakes	6 fl. oz.	90	0.0	0	0.0
Chilled, Sunkist	6 fl. oz.	76	0.3	0	3.5

■ Contains less than 20% fat

Item	PORTION	CAL-ORIES	FAT GRAMS	CHOLES-TEROL	% OF FAT
Frozen, Citrus Hill, prepared					
Regular	6 fl. oz.	90	0.1	0	1.0
Lite	6 fl. oz.	60	0.1	0	1.5
Orange/grape, canned	½ cup	53	0.1	0	1.7
Orange-pineapple-banana, canned, Land O'Lakes	6 fl. oz.	100	0.0	0	0.0
Papaya, canned	½ cup	77	0.1	0	1.1
Peach juice, canned, Smucker's	6 fl. oz.	90	0.0	0	0.0
Pineapple					
Canned, un-sweetened, Town House	6 fl. oz.	100	0.0	0	0.0
Frozen, unsweet-ened, Dole, prepared	6 fl. oz.	90	0.0	0	0.0
Pineapple/grape, canned	½ cup	53	0.1	0	1.7
Pineapple/grapefruit, fro-zen, Dole, prepared	6 fl. oz.	90	0.0	0	0.0
Pineapple/orange, canned, Ardmore Farms	6 fl. oz.	102	0.1	0	0.9
Prune, canned, Lady Betty	6 fl. oz.	130	0.0	0	0.0
Raspberry, red, canned, Smucker's	6 fl. oz.	90	0.0	0	0.0
Tangerine, un-sweetened, canned	½ cup	53	0.2	0	3.4

■ Contains less than 20% fat

Item	PORTION	CALORIES	FAT GRAMS	CHOLESTEROL	% OF FAT
Tomato juice, canned					
Regular, Ardmore Farms	6 fl. oz.	36	0.1	0	2.5
Dietetic, Hunt's	6 fl. oz.	30	0.1	0	3.0
Vegetable					
Cocktail, canned, Smucker's	6 fl. oz.	44	0.1	0	2.0
V-8, regular or low salt	6 fl. oz.	35	0.1	0	2.6
■Kool-Aid					
Canned, KA Koolers					
Cherry or mountain-berry punch	8.45 fl. oz.	142	0.1	0	0.6
Grape	8.45 fl. oz.	136	0.1	0	0.7
Orange	8.45 fl. oz.	115	0.1	0	0.8
Mix					
Pre-sweetened					
Grape	8 fl. oz.	80	0.0	0	0.0
Rainbow punch	8 fl. oz.	84	0.0	0	0.0
Sugar to be added	8 fl. oz.	98	0.0	0	0.0
Sugar-free, dietetic, grape	8 fl. oz.	3	0.0	0	0.0
■Lemonade					
Canned					
Hi-C	8.45 fl. oz.	109	0.1	0	0.8
Kool-Aid Koolers	8.45 fl. oz.	120	0.0	0	0.0
Frozen, prepared, Country Time	8 fl. oz.	96	0.02	0	0.2
Mix, prepared					
Regular, 4C	8 fl. oz.	80	0.0	0	0.0

■ Contains less than 20% fat   6

Item	PORTION	CAL-ORIES	FAT GRAMS	CHOLES-TEROL	% OF FAT
Dietetic, Country Time	8 fl. oz.	4	0.0	0	0.0
■Lemonade punch, mix, Country Time, prepared	8 fl. oz.	82	0.0	0	0.0
■Lemon-limeade, mix, dietetic, Crystal Light, prepared	8 fl. oz.	4	0.0	0	0.0
■Limeade, frozen, dilute	8 fl. oz.	101	0.0	0	0.0
Milk (See Dairy & Dairy Products, milk)					
■Nectar, canned					
Apple, Libby's	6 fl. oz.	100	0.0	0	0.0
Apricot, Town House	6 fl. oz.	100	0.0	0	0.0
Banana, Libby's	6 fl. oz.	110	0.0	0	0.0
Peach, Ardmore Farms	6 fl. oz.	90	0.0	0	0.1
■Orange drink					
Canned, Ardmore Farms	6 fl. oz.	86	0.0	0	0.0
Mix, prepared					
Regular, Funny Face	6 fl. oz.	66	0.0	0	0.0
Dietetic, Crystal Light	6 fl. oz.	4	0.0	0	0.0
■Peach drink, canned, Hi-C	6 fl. oz.	101	0.01	0	0.0
■Punch drink, canned, Minute Maid	8.45 fl. oz.	131	0.1	0	0.7
■Seltzer, unsweetened	12 fl. oz.	0	0.0	0	0.0
■Soda					
Club, Shasta	12 fl. oz.	0	0.0	0	0.0
Cream, Canada Dry	12 fl. oz.	194	0.0	0	0.0
Ginger ale, Schweppes	12 fl. oz.	130	0.0	0	0.0

Item	PORTION	CAL-ORIES	FAT GRAMS	CHOLES-TEROL	% OF FAT
Grape, Hi-C	12 fl. oz.	158	0.0	0	0.0
Lemon sour, Schweppes	12 fl. oz.	158	0.0	0	0.0
Orange, Fanta	12 fl. oz.	176	0.0	0	0.0
Root beer, Fanta	12 fl. oz.	156	0.0	0	0.0
7Up	12 fl. oz.	144	0.0	0	0.0
Soy Drinks					
Ah Soy					
■ Carob	6 fl. oz.	160	3.0	0	16.8
Vanilla	6 fl. oz.	160	5.0	0	28.1
■Tang					
Canned, Fruit Box					
Cherry or straw-berry	8.45 fl. oz.	121	0.1	0	0.7
Orange	8.45 fl. oz.	127	0.1	0	0.7
Mix, prepared, orange					
Sweetened	6 fl. oz.	86	0.1	0	1.0
Dietetic	6 fl. oz.	5	0.01	0	1.8
■Tea, brewed					
Plain	6 fl. oz.	2	0.0	0	0.0
Plain, instant	6 fl. oz.	2	0.0	0	0.0
Flavored, Celestial Seasonings					
Bavarian choco-late orange	6 fl. oz.	7	0.0	0	0.0
Irish cream mist	6 fl. oz.	3	0.0	0	0.0
Herb, Celestial Seasonings					
Almond sunset	6 fl. oz.	3	0.0	0	0.0
Lemon zinger	6 fl. oz.	4	0.0	0	0.0
Roastaroma	6 fl. oz.	11	0.1	0	8.2
■Tea, iced					
Canned, sweet-ened, Johanna Farms Ssips	8.45 fl. oz.	100	0.0	0	0.0
Mix, prepared					
Sugar & lemon flavored, 4C	8 fl. oz.	90	0.0	0	0.0

Item	PORTION	CAL-ORIES	FAT GRAMS	CHOLES-TEROL	% OF FAT
Dietetic, Crystal Light	8 fl. oz.	3	0.0	0	0.0
■Tonic water or quinine, Canada Dry	12 fl. oz.	136	0.0	0	0.0
■Wild berry drink, canned, Hi-C	6 fl. oz.	92	0.1	0	1.0

BREADS & BREADSTUFFS

Item	PORTION	CAL-ORIES	FAT GRAMS	CHOLES-TEROL	% OF FAT
■Bagels					
Egg					
Lender's	1	190	2.0	5	9.5
Sara Lee	1	210	1.0	–	4.3
Onion					
Lender's	1	179	1.0	0	5.0
Sara Lee	1	210	1.0	–	4.3
Plain	1	161	1.5	–	8.4
Lender's	1	179	1.0	0	5.0
Raisin & Honey Lender's	1	190	1.0	0	4.7
■Bialy	1	80	0.0	0	0.0
Biscuits					
Homemade	1	127	6.4	2	45.3
Mix, made w/milk	1-oz. piece	91	2.6	0	25.7
Baking powder, 1869 Brand	1	100	5.0	0	45.0
Buttermilk, Pillsbury					
■ Ballard Ovenready	1	50	1.0	0	18.0
1869 Brand	1	100	5.0	0	45.0
Hungry Jack					
■ Extra rich	1	50	1.0	0	18.0
Fluffy	1	90	4.0	5	40.0

■ Contains less than 20% fat   9

Item	PORTION	CAL-ORIES	FAT GRAMS	CHOLES-TEROL	% OF FAT
Butter Tastin', 1869 Brand	1	100	5.0	0	45.0
Flaky, Pillsbury Hungry Jack					
Regular	1	80	4.0	0	45.0
Honey	1	90	4.0	0	40.0
Heat 'n Eat, Pillsbury Premium	1	140	7.5	–	48.2
■Homestyle, Mrs. Wright's	1	50	0.7	–	12.6
Oat bran, Roman Meal	1	130	5.0	–	34.6
Southern, Pillsbury Big Country	1	100	4.0	–	36.0
X-Lite, Pillsbury	1	60	1.5	–	22.5

Breads

Item	PORTION	CAL-ORIES	FAT GRAMS	CHOLES-TEROL	% OF FAT
■Apple cinnamon, Pritikin	1 slice	80	1.0	3	11.2
■Black, Mrs. Wright's	1 slice	60	1.0	–	15.0
Bran, Roman Meal					
■ 5 Bran	1 slice	65	1.1	0	15.2
■ Oat	1 slice	42	0.5	0	10.7
Rice	1 slice	71	1.8	0	22.8
■Brown, Boston, canned	1 slice	93	0.5	0	4.8
Cinnamon, Pepper-idge Farm	1 slice	90	3.0	0	30.0
Cornbread, 2″ × 2.5″	1 slice	147	4.7	26	28.8
■French					
Du Jour	1 slice	70	1.0	0	12.8
Vienna	1 slice	73	0.5	1	6.5
Garlic, Arnold	1 slice	80	3.0	–	33.7
■Granola bran, Mrs. Wright's Grainbelt	1 slice	140	2.0	0	12.8
■Hi-fibre, Monk's	1 slice	50	1.0	0	18.0

■ Contains less than 20% fat

Item	PORTION	CAL-ORIES	FAT GRAMS	CHOLES-TEROL	% OF FAT
■Honey & molasses graham, Mrs. Wright's Grainbelt	1 slice	100	1.0	0	9.0
Honey wheatberry, Arnold	1 slice	80	2.0	5	22.5
■Italian					
Arnold Francisco	1 slice	70	1.0	–	12.9
Pepperidge Farm, brown & serve, Hearth	1-oz. piece	80	1.0	0	11.2
Low sodium, Eddy's	1 slice	80	2.0	–	22.5
■Multi-grain, Arnold Milk & Honey	1 slice	70	1.0	–	12.9
■Oat, Weight Watchers	1 slice	39	0.4	0	9.2
■Oat bran, Roman Meal	1 slice	69	1.1	0	14.3
Oatmeal, Pepperidge Farm					
■ Regular	1 slice	90	1.0	–	10.0
■ Light	1 slice	45	0.0	0	0.0
Very thin sliced	1 slice	40	1.0	0	22.5
■Onion dill, Pritikin	1 slice	70	1.0	–	12.9
Pita, Thomas' Sahara					
Plain	2-oz. piece	160	1.0	–	5.6
Whole wheat	2-oz. piece	150	2.0	–	11.2
■Pumpernickel, Pepperidge Farm					
Family	1 slice	80	1.0	–	11.2
Party	1 slice	15	0.2	–	0.1
■Raisin					
Pritikin	1 slice	70	1.0	–	12.9
Sunmaid, Arnold	1 slice	80	1.0	–	11.2
Weight Watchers	1 slice	49	0.6	0	11.0
■Rye					
Levy's	1 slice	80	1.0	0	11.2

Item	PORTION	CAL-ORIES	FAT GRAMS	CHOLES-TEROL	% OF FAT
Pepperidge Farm					
Dijon, hearty	1 slice	70	1.0	0	12.8
Family	1 slice	80	1.0	0	11.2
Pritikin	1 slice	70	1.0	–	12.9
■7-Grain, Roman Meal					
Regular	1 slice	66	0.7	0	9.5
Light	1 slice	40	0.4	0	9.0
■Sourdough	1 slice	139	1.1	0	7.1
Sun grain, Roman Meal	1 slice	70	1.6	0	20.6
■Wheat					
Regular, Pepperidge Farm					
Family	1 slice	70	1.0	0	12.9
Light	1 slice	45	0.0	0	0.0
Cracked, Roman Meal	1 slice	67	0.9	0	12.1
■Wheatberry, Roman Meal					
Regular	1 slice	64	0.7	0	9.8
Light	1 slice	39	0.2	0	4.6
■White					
Arnold, brick oven (1 lb. loaf)	1 slice	60	1.0	–	15.0
Homepride, buttertop	1 slice	74	1.1	1	13.4
Roman Meal, light	1 slice	40	0.2	0	4.5
■White, with butter-milk, Wonder	1 slice	72	1.1	1	13.7
■Whole grain, Roman Meal	1 slice	63	0.9	0	12.9
■Whole wheat					
Pepperidge Farm, thin slice	1 slice	60	1.0	0	15.0
Pritikin	1 slice	70	1.0	0	12.8
Breads, Sweetened					
Coffeecake	2 oz.	198	8.9	48	40.5

Item	PORTION	CALORIES	FAT GRAMS	CHOLESTEROL	% OF FAT
Danish					
Apple, Dolly Madison	1	240	13.0	–	48.7
Caramel w/nuts, Pillsbury	1	160	8.0	5	45.0
Cheese, cream, Dolly Madison	1	380	20.0	–	47.4
Donut					
Cake	1	156	7.4	24	42.7
Yeast-leavened	1	166	10.7	10	58.0
Dolly Madison					
Regular, chocolate coated	1	150	8.0	–	48.0
Dunkin' Stix	1	210	15.0	–	64.3
Jumbo, plain	1	190	10.0	–	47.4
Honey Bun, Hostess	1	579	33.7	34	52.4
Sweet roll					
Cinnamon w/icing, refrigerated dough	1	280	11.0	–	35.4
Cinnamon, Sara Lee	1	320	15.0	–	42.2
Plain	1	162	5.8	27	32.2
Muffins					
Plain					
Homemade	1	131	4.8	18	33.0
Commercial	1	118	4.0	21	30.5
Apple Spice					
■ Healthy Choice	1	130	1.0	0	6.9
Sara Lee Hearty Fruit	1	220	8.0	–	32.7
Weight Watchers	1 (2.5 oz.)	160	5.0	0	28.1
Banana Nut					
Harts	1 (1.5 oz.)	148	4.6	5	27.9
Dunkin' Donuts	1 (1.31 oz.)	327	12.0	–	33.0

■ Contains less than 20% fat   13

Item	PORTION	CAL-ORIES	FAT GRAMS	CHOLES-TEROL	% OF FAT
■ Pepperidge Farm	1	250	5.0	–	18.0
Weight Watchers	1	170	5.0	10	26.5
Blueberry					
Dunkin' Donuts	1	280	8.0	30	25.7
■ Hostess, Low Fat	1 (1.25 oz.)	100	1.0	0	9.0
Mr. Donut	1 (1.35 oz.)	343	13.0	–	34.1
Pepperidge Farm	1	170	7.0	25	37.1
Sara Lee	1 (2.5 oz.)	200	8.0	0	36.0
■ Sara Lee Free & Light	1	120	0.0	0	0.0
Weight Watchers	1	170	5.0	10	26.5
Blueberry/Strawberry, Betty Crocker	1	180	6.0	–	30.0
■Bran	1	140	2.6	30	16.7
Carrot nut, Betty Crocker	1	150	5.0	25	30.0
Chocolate chip, Betty Crocker					
Regular	1	150	5.0	20	30.0
No cholesterol recipe	1	140	5.0	0	32.1
Cinnamon swirl, Duncan Hines, bakery style	1	195	5.4	0	24.9
Corn					
Pepperidge Farm	1	180	7.0	30	35.0
Sara Lee	1	460	24.0	–	47.0
■English Muffin					
Cinnamon Raisin-Chip, Pepperidge Farm	1	150	2.0	–	12.0
Plain	1	182	3.6	32	17.8
Pritikin	1	135	2.0	0	13.3
Thomas'	1	130	1.4	0	9.7
■ Wolferman's De Luxe	1	220	2.0	0	8.2

■ Contains less than 20% fat   14

Item	PORTION	CAL-ORIES	FAT GRAMS	CHOLES-TEROL	% OF FAT
■ Wonder	1	120	1.0	0	7.5
Sourdough, Thomas'	1	120	1.0	0	7.5
Fruit/Fiber, Entenmann's	1 (2.5 oz.)	248	9.0	–	32.7
■Granola, Mrs. Wright's	1	150	1.0	0	6.0
Honey bran, Gold Medal	1	170	6.0	–	31.8
Honey Raisin, Entenmann's	1 (2.5 oz.)	248	9.0	–	32.7
Oat Bran					
* Basic	1	126	2.9	–	20.7
Mr. Donut	1 (4.4 oz.)	436	12.0	–	24.8
Pepperidge Farm, w/apple, cholesterol free	1	190	7.0	0	33.1
Sara Lee	1 (2.5 oz.)	220	8.0	–	32.7
Sara Lee	1	330	9.0	–	24.5
Raisin bran, Dunkin' Donuts	1 (3.7 oz.)	310	9.0	15	26.1
Rolls					
Apple, Dolly Madison	1	180	4.0	–	20.0
■Blunt, Mrs. Wright's	1	150	2.0	–	12.0
Brown & serve, Roman Meal	1	72	1.8	0	22.5
■Country, Pepperidge Farm	1	50	1.0	0	18.0
Crescent					
Mrs. Wright's	1	95	4.0	–	37.9
Pillsbury	1	95	5.0	–	47.4
Croissant					
Regular	1	272	17.3	47	57.2
Butter, petite, Sara Lee	1	120	6.0	–	45.0

Item	PORTION	CAL-ORIES	FAT GRAMS	CHOLES-TEROL	% OF FAT
Merico Lite Fluff	1	95	4.0	–	37.9
Mrs. Wright's	1	95	4.0	–	37.9
Pepperidge Farm	1	170	7.0	0	37.1
Sara Lee	1	105	5.9	–	50.6
■Deli Krisp, Mrs. Wright's	1	120	2.0	–	15.0
Dinner					
Mrs. Wright's, regular	1	47	2.0	–	38.3
Pillsbury Butterflake	1	140	5	–	30.0
■ Roman Meal	1	75	1.5	0	18.0
Finger, Pepperidge Farm	1	50	2.0	3	36.0
French					
■ Mrs. Wright's	1	160	3.0	–	16.9
■ Pepperidge Farm	1	100	1.0	0	9.0
■Hamburger bun					
Mrs. Wright's					
Regular	1	190	3.0	0	14.2
Lite	1	80	1.0	0	11.2
Onion	1	130	2.0	0	13.8
Wheat, crushed, giant	1	170	2.0	0	10.6
Roman Meal	1	122	2.5	0	18.4
■Hard	1	156	1.6	2	9.2
Hoagie, Pepperidge Farm	1	210	5.0	0	21.4
Homestyle, Rich's	1	75	2.0	–	24.0
Hot dog bun					
■ Mrs. Wright's, wheat, crushed	1	110	1.0	0	8.2
Pepperidge Farm					
■ Regular	1	140	3.0	0	19.3
Dijon	1	160	5.0	0	28.1
■Hot roll, Pillsbury, prepared	1	120	2.0	–	15.0

Item	PORTION	CAL-ORIES	FAT GRAMS	CHOLES-TEROL	% OF FAT
■Italian, crusty, Du Jour	1	80	1.0	0	11.2
■Kaiser, sandwich, Sara Lee	1	161	3.1	–	17.3
Old-fashioned, Pepperidge Farm	1	50	2.0	5	36.0
■Parker House, Pepperidge Farm	1	60	1.0	5	15.0
Potato, Pepperidge Farm, hearty classic	1	90	3.0	0	30.0
■Rye, light, Sara Lee	1	79	0.9	–	10.2
■Sourdough					
Mrs. Wright's	1	190	2.0	0	9.5
Pioneer	1	105	0.7	0	6.0
■Steak, Butternut	1 (1 oz.)	80	1.0	–	11.2
Whole wheat	1	72	1.8	9	22.5
Stuffing					
■Apple & raisin, Pepperidge Farm	1 oz.	110	1.0	–	8.2
Bread, from mix, w/water, fat	½ cup	245	15.2	45	55.8
Bread, prepared, no salt	½ cup	166	8.0	21	43.4
Chicken, from mix, prepared					
Bell's	½ cup	224	13.0	–	52.2
Town House	½ cup	180	9.0	–	45.0
Cornbread					
■ Pepperidge Farm, mix	1 oz.	110	1.0	–	8.2
Town House, mix, prepared	½ cup	170	8.0	–	42.3
Herb, from mix, prepared, Betty Crocker	½ cup	190	9.0	–	42.6
Stove Top, mix	½ cup	176	9.0	21	46.0

■ Contains less than 20% fat   17

Item	PORTION	CAL-ORIES	FAT GRAMS	CHOLES-TEROL	% OF FAT
■Wild rice, Golden Grain	1 oz.	108	1.1	0	9.2
Wild rice & mushroom, Pepperidge Farm	1 oz.	130	5.0	–	34.6

Other Breadstuffs
■Breadcrumbs

Item	PORTION	CAL-ORIES	FAT GRAMS	CHOLES-TEROL	% OF FAT
Fresh, made from white bread	1 tb.	25	0.3	–	10.8
4 C, plain or seasoned	1 tb.	35	0.7	–	18.0
Progresso, Italian style	1 tb.	30	0.0	0	0.0

Breadsticks
Refrigerated

Item	PORTION	CAL-ORIES	FAT GRAMS	CHOLES-TEROL	% OF FAT
■ Pillsbury, soft	1	100	17.0	0	18.0
Roman Meal	1	117	3.9	0	30.0

Plain

Item	PORTION	CAL-ORIES	FAT GRAMS	CHOLES-TEROL	% OF FAT
Keebler	1	17	0.5	–	26.5
Stella D'Oro	1	40	1.0	0	22.5
Sesame, Stella D'Oro	1	50	2.0	0	36.0
■Corn flake crumbs	1 oz.	110	0.1	0	0.8
Corn fritters	1	151	8.6	35	51.2
Crepe, plain shell	1	80	2.7	71	30.4

Croutons

Item	PORTION	CAL-ORIES	FAT GRAMS	CHOLES-TEROL	% OF FAT
■ Kellogg's Croutettes	⅔ cup	70	0.0	–	0.0

Pepperidge Farm

Item	PORTION	CAL-ORIES	FAT GRAMS	CHOLES-TEROL	% OF FAT
Cheddar & romano cheese	½ oz.	60	2.0	0	30.0
Cheese & garlic or seasoned	½ oz.	70	3.0	0	38.6
■Egg Roll Wrapper	1	20	0	0	0.0
Hush Puppies	1	51	2.3	27	40.6

■ Contains less than 20% fat

Item	PORTION	CAL-ORIES	FAT GRAMS	CHOLES-TEROL	% OF FAT
Popover, homemade w/enriched flour	1	90	3.6	59	36.0
■Tortilla					
Corn, Old El Paso	1	60	1.0	–	15.0
Flour, Old El Paso	1	150	3.0	–	18.0
Whole wheat, large	1	98	0.9	0	8.3
■Tostada or Taco Shell					
Old El Paso	1	60	3.0	0	45.0
■Zwieback	1	30	0.6	1	18.0

BREAKFAST FOODS

Cereal
Item	PORTION	CAL-ORIES	FAT GRAMS	CHOLES-TEROL	% OF FAT
■All Bran					
Plain	⅓ cup	70	1.0	0	12.9
W/extra fiber	½ cup	50	0.0	0	0.0
■Alpha-Bits	1 cup	111	0.6	0	4.8
■Apple Jacks	1 cup	110	0.1	0	0.8
▓Basic 4, General Mills	¾ cup	130	2.0	0	13.0
■Batman	1 cup	110	1.0	0	9.0
■Bigg Mixx, plain	½ cup	110	2.0	0	16.4
■Blueberry Squares, Kellogg's	⅔ cup	90	0.0	0	0.0
■Body Buddies	1 cup	110	1.0	0	8.2
■Breakfast With Barbie	1 cup	110	1.0	0	8.2
Bran					
■ Oat, dry, uncooked, Quaker	1 oz.	109	2.2	0	18.1
■ Raisin, Kellogg's	1 cup	153	1.0	0	5.8
■ Wheat, crude	1 oz.	61	1.2	0	17.7
■ Whole wheat, prepared, Quaker	1 cup	138	0.9	0	5.8
■40% Bran Flakes, Kellogg's	1 cup	127	0.7	0	4.9
■100% Bran, Kellogg's	1 cup	178	3.3	0	16.6
■Bran Buds	1 cup	217	2.0	0	8.2

■ Contains less than 20% fat   19

Item	PORTION	CAL-ORIES	FAT GRAMS	CHOLES-TEROL	% OF FAT
■Bran Chex, Ralston Purina	1 cup	156	1.3	0	7.5
■Cap 'N Crunch	1 cup	151	2.1	0	12.5
■Cheerios, plain	1 cup	89	1.5	0	15.1
Honey Nut	1 cup	125	0.7	0	5.0
■ Apple cinnamon	1 oz.	110	2.0	0	16.4
■ Honey nut	1 oz.	110	1.0	0	8.2
■ Multi-grain	1 oz.	100	1.0	0	9.0
Cinnamon Toast Crunch, General Mills	1 cup	160	4.0	0	22.5
■Cocoa Puffs, General Mills	1 cup	110	0.5	0	4.1
■Coco Wheats, Little Crow					
Regular	1 tb.	43	0.3	0	6.3
Instant	1¼ oz.	130	0.0	0	0.0
■Common Sense Oat Bran	1 oz.	100	1.0	0	9.0
■Corn Chex, Ralston Purina	1 oz.	111	0.1	0	0.8
■Corn Flakes, Kellogg's					
Plain	1 cup	88	0.1	0	1.0
Sugar Frosted	1 cup	133	0.1	0	0.6
■Cornmeal, degermed, yellow	1 cup	104	0.5	0	4.3
■Corn Pops	1 pkt.	81	0.1	0	1.1
Cracklin' Bran	1 cup	229	8.8	0	34.5
■Cream of Wheat					
Instant, dry, Nabisco	1 oz.	100	0.0	0	0
Prepared	1 cup	104	0.5	0	4.3
■Crispix, Kellogg's	1 cup	110	0.0	0	0.0
■Crisp rice					
Crisp & Crackling Rice	1 cup	108	0.3	0	2.5
Safeway	1 cup	110	0.0	0	0.0
■Crispy Critters, Post	1 cup	110	0.0	0	0.0

■ Contains less than 20% fat   20

Item	PORTION	CAL-ORIES	FAT GRAMS	CHOLES-TEROL	% OF FAT
■Crispy Wheats 'N Raisins, General Mills	¾ cup	110	1.0	0	8.2
C W Post, plain	⅓ cup	144	5.0	0	31.2
■Farina, cooked	1 cup	116	0.2	0	1.5
■Fiber One, General Mills	½ cup	60	1.0	0	15.0
■Fruit/Fiber, Post					
Apple/cinnamon	1 cup	177	0.7	0	3.5
Raisins/dates/ walnut	1 cup	176	1.4	0	7.1
■Froot Loops	1 cup	111	0.5	0	4.0
■Garfield and Friends, General Mills	.9 oz.	100	2.0	–	18.0
■Golden Grahams Granola	1 cup	150	1.4	0	8.4
Cinnamon/raisin, Nature Valley	⅓ cup	160	5.6	0	31.5
■ Fat free, Health Valley	1 oz.	90	0.0	0	0.0
*■ Homemade serving	½ cup	208	2.2	1	9.5
■Grape-nuts	⅓ cup	135	0.2	0	1.3
■Grape-nuts flakes	1 cup	116	0.4	0	3.1
■Grits					
Corn, yellow, cooked	1 cup	145	0.5	0	3.1
Instant, dry, Quaker	1 oz.	79	0.2	0	2.2
■Fiberwise, Kellogg's	1 oz.	90	1.0	0	10.0
■Honeycomb, crunch, Post	1⅓ cups	110	0.5	0	4.1
■Honey Smacks, Kellogg's	¾ cup	110	0.5	0	4.1
■Just Right, with fiber nuggets	⅔ cup	100	0.5	0	4.5
■Kaboom, General Mills	1 cup	110	0.5	0	4.1

■ Contains less than 20% fat   21   * See page xxxii

Item	PORTION	CAL-ORIES	FAT GRAMS	CHOLES-TEROL	% OF FAT
■Kasli, Hodgson Mills	⅔ cup	236	1.3	0	4.9
■Kix	1 cup	74	0.4	0	4.8
■Life, plain or cinnamon	1 cup	172	2.7	0	14.1
■Lucky Charms	1 cup	110	1.2	0	9.8
■Malt-O-Meal					
Uncooked	1 oz.	100	0.0	0	0.0
Cooked					
Plain	1 cup	122	0.2	0	1.4
Chocolate	1 cup	122	0.2	0	1.4
■Marshmallow Krispies	1¼ cups	140	0.0	0	0.0
■Most	1 cup	175	0.6	0	3.0
■Muesli, Familia	½ cup	424	6.0	0	12.7
■Müeslix, crispy blend, Kellogg's	⅔ cup	160	2.0	0	11.2
Natural					
Heartland, raisin	¼ cup	130	4.0	–	27.7
Nature Valley, toasted oat	⅓ cup	130	5.0	0	34.6
■Multi-Grain, Quaker	½ cup	130	1.5	0	10.0
■Nintendo Cereal System, Ralston-Purina	1 cup	110	1.0	0	8.2
■Nut & Honey Crunch, Kellogg's	⅔ cup	110	1.0	0	8.2
■Nutri-Grain					
Almond-raisin	1 cup	210	3.0	0	12.9
Raisin-bran	1 cup	130	1.0	0	6.9
Wheat	1 cup	150	0.0	0	0.0
■Oat & wheat, cooked	1 cup	159	2.0	0	11.3
Oatbake, Kellogg's	⅓ cup	110	3.0	0	24.5
■Oat Bran O's,					
Plain, Health Valley	1 cup	120	2.7	0	20.2
Fruit & nut, Health Valley	1 cup	120	2.7	0	20.2

■ Contains less than 20% fat   22

Item	PORTION	CAL-ORIES	FAT GRAMS	CHOLES-TEROL	% OF FAT
■Oatios	1 cup	86	0.8	0	8.3
■Oat Flakes, Post	1 oz.	110	1.0	0	8.0
■Oatmeal, cooked	1 cup	145	2.3	0	14.2
■ Quaker	1 cup	94	2.0	0	19.1
■ High Fiber, Smart Beat	1 cup	140	3.0	0	19.0
■Oatmeal, instant					
Plain, Quaker	1 pkt.	100	2.0	0	14.0
W/cinnamon spice, Quaker	1 pkt.	118	1.5	0	11.0
■Oats & Fiber, H-O, dry					
Boxed	⅓ cup	100	2.0	0	18.0
Packet, raisin & bran	1 pkt.	150	2.0	0	12.0
■Pebbles, Post	⅞ cup	113	1.0	0	8.0
■Product 19	1 cup	100	0.2	0	1.4
■Rice, puffed	1 oz.	114	0.1	0	0.7
■Rice Chex, Ralston Purina	1 cup	100	0.1	0	0.9
■Rice Krinkles, frosted	1 cup	125	0.1	0	0.7
■Rice Krispies	1 cup	112	0.2	0	1.6
Roman Meal, hot Regular					
■ Original, plain	⅓ cup	82	0.5	0	5.5
Multi-bran w/cinnamon & apples	⅓ cup	112	2.8	0	22.5
Instant w/oats, wheat, honey, coconut & almond	⅓ cup	154	5.6	0	32.7
■7 Grain, w/raisins, Health Valley	⅓ cup	146	1.3	0	8.0
■Seven Grain, cooked, Arrowhead Mills	1 oz.	100	1.0	0	9.0
■Special K, Kellogg's	1 cup	110	0.1	0	1.0

■ Contains less than 20% fat

Item	PORTION	CAL-ORIES	FAT GRAMS	CHOLES-TEROL	% OF FAT
■Sugar Frosted Flakes, Kellogg's	1 cup	133	0.1	0	0.6
■Sugar Puffs, Malt-O-Meal	1 cup	109	0.4	0	3.3
■Team	1 cup	164	0.7	0	3.8
■Teenage Mutant Ninja Turtles, Ralston Purina	1 cup	110	0.0	0	0.0
■Toasty O's, Malt-O-Meal, plain	1¼ cups	107	1.9	0	16.0
■Tootie Fruities, Malt-O-Meal	1 cup	113	1.1	0	8.8
■Total					
Regular or corn	1 cup	110	1.0	0	8.2
Raisin bran	1 cup	140	1.0	0	6.4
■Trix	1 oz.	109	0.4	0	3.3
■Wheat, shredded					
Spoonsize	1 cup	153	0.9	0	5.2
'N Bran, Nabisco	1 cup	163	1.5	0	8.2
W/Oat Bran	1 oz.	100	1.0	0	9.0
■Wheat Chex, Ralston Purina	1 cup	169	1.1	0	5.8
■Wheat flakes, PEP, Kellogg's	1 cup	117	0.3	0	2.3
Wheat germ					
Kretschmer	1 oz.	110	3.0	0	24.5
Toasted	1 oz.	108	3.0	0	25.0
■Wheat Hearts, dry, hot, General Mills	1 tb.	85	0.8	0	8.5
■Wheatena, hot	1 oz.	100	1.0	0	9.0
■Wheaties	1 cup	100	0.5	0	4.5
■Wheat, puffed					
Malt-O-Meal	1 cup	53	0.4	0	6.8
Post	⅞ cup	104	0.2	0	1.7

Item	PORTION	CAL-ORIES	FAT GRAMS	CHOLES-TEROL	% OF FAT
Pancakes					
* Homemade, buckwheat	2	177	5.1	123	25.9
Mix, prepared					
Plain					
Aunt Jemima, original	2	134	5.4	–	36.3
■ Bisquick Shake 'N Pour	2	174	3.4	0	17.6
■ Ester, dietetic	2	66	0.0	0	0.0
Hungry Jack					
Extra Lights					
Regular	2	140	4.6	–	29.6
■ Complete	2	126	1.4	–	10.0
Panshakes	2	186	4.0	–	21.7
■ Apple cinnamon, Bisquick					
Shake 'N Pour	2	180	3.4	0	17.0
Blueberry					
■ FastShake, Little Crow	2	125	1.5	1	10.8
Hungry Jack	2	214	10.0	–	42.1
■ Butter flavor, Mrs. Butterworth's, complete	2	126	2.0	–	14.3
■ Buttermilk					
Betty Crocker, complete	2	140	2.0	–	12.6
Gold Medal	2	200	4.0	–	18.0
■ Oat bran, Bisquick Shake 'N Pour	2	160	2.6	0	14.6
Frozen					
■ Aunt Jemima					
Buttermilk	3½ oz.	210	3.0	20	12.8
Lite	3½ oz.	140	3.0	–	19.3
Lite w/lite syrup	6 oz.	260	3.0	–	10.4
Downyflake					
Plain	3	280	9.0	–	28.9

■ Contains less than 20% fat   25   * See page xxxii

Item	PORTION	CAL-ORIES	FAT GRAMS	CHOLES-TEROL	% OF FAT
Blueberry	3	280	9.0	–	28.9
Great Starts, Swanson					
W/bacon	1 (4.5 oz.)	400	20.0	–	45.0
& sausage	1 (6 oz.)	460	22.0	–	43.0
Silver dollar, & sausage	1 (3¾ oz.)	310	14.0	–	40.6
Whole wheat, w/lite links	1 (5.5 oz.)	350	16.0	–	41.1
■ Pillsbury, microwave					
Blueberry	2	166	2.6	–	14.1
Wheat, harvest	2	160	2.6	–	14.6
■ Weight Watchers					
w/blueberry topping	4.8 oz.	200	4.0	10	18.0
Buttermilk	2½ oz.	140	3.0	10	19.3
w/strawberry topping	4¾ oz.	230	4.0	10	15.6
■Frozen, batter, Aunt Jemima, regular	2	180	1.4	–	7.0

Waffles

Item	PORTION	CAL-ORIES	FAT GRAMS	CHOLES-TEROL	% OF FAT
* Homemade, oat bran	1	174	4.1	3	21.2
Frozen					
Plain					
Eggo, homestyle	1	120	5.0	–	37.5
Great Starts, Swanson, w/bacon	1 (2.2 oz.)	230	14.0	–	54.8
Nutri-Grain, Eggo	1	130	5.0	0	34.6
Apple cinnamon, Aunt Jemima	1	90	3.0	–	30.0
Belgian					
Great Starts, Swanson					
& sausage	1 (2.85 oz.)	280	19.0	–	61.1

Item	PORTION	CAL-ORIES	FAT GRAMS	CHOLES-TEROL	% OF FAT
& strawber-ries, w/sausage	1 (3.5 oz.)	210	8.0	–	34.3
Weight Watchers Blueberry	1 (1.5 oz.)	120	4.0	5	30.0
Aunt Jemima	2½ oz.	180	5.0	5	25.0
Downyflake	1	90	2.0	0	20.0
Eggo	1	130	5.0	–	34.6
Downy Flake	2	120	3.0	–	22.4
Multi-bran, Nutri-Grain	2.9 oz.	240	10.0	–	37.5
Nut & honey, Eggo	2.8 oz.	260	12.0	–	41.5
Oat bran, plain, Common Sense, Eggo	1	110	4.0	0	32.7
Belgian Chef	2.4 oz.	160	6.0	–	33.7
Raisin & bran, Nutri-Grain, Eggo	1	130	5.0	0	34.6
■ Special K, Eggo	1	80	0.0	0	0.0

**Other Breakfast Foods
(see also Breads, Sweet;
Eggs, Egg Dishes & Egg Substitutes)**

Item	PORTION	CAL-ORIES	FAT GRAMS	CHOLES-TEROL	% OF FAT
Breakfast bar, choco-late chip, Carna-tion	1	198	10.6	0	48.1
*■Burrito, breakfast	1	187	3.8	0	18.3
Cereal Bar					
Common Sense oat bran w/raspberry filling	1	170	6.0	0	31.8
Corn flakes w/mixed berry filling	1	170	7.0	0	37.1
Nutri-Grain, blue-berry	1	180	8.0	0	40.0

■ Contains less than 20% fat   27   * See page xxxii

Item	PORTION	CAL-ORIES	FAT GRAMS	CHOLES-TEROL	% OF FAT
Rice Krispies w/almonds	1	130	6.0	0	41.5
English muffin					
■ W/turkey or ham, Healthy Choice	1	200	3.0	20	13.5
Sandwich, Weight Watchers	1	230	8.0	160	31.3
French toast, frozen					
Aunt Jemima, cinnamon swirl, thick slice	1	110	3.5	45	28.6
Great Starts, Swanson					
Cinnamon swirl, w/sausage	1 (5.5 oz.)	390	21.0	–	48.5
Mini, w/sausage	1 (2.5 oz.)	190	9.0	–	42.6
Oatmeal, w/lite links	1 (4.6 oz.)	310	13.0	–	37.7
■Instant breakfast, dry, Carnation					
Chocolate	1 env.	130	0.9	3	6.2
Strawberry	1 env.	130	0.2	2	1.3
Vanilla	1 env.	130	0.2	2	1.3
■Omelet, turkey sausage, Healthy Choice	1	210	4.0	20	17.0
Pop Tarts, Kellogg's					
Regular, blueberry Frosted	1	210	6.0	0	25.7
Brown sugar	1	210	7.0	0	30.0
Concord grape	1	200	6.0	0	27.0
Toaster Tarts, Pepperidge Farm, Cheese	1	190	10.0	10	47.4

Item	PORTION	CAL-ORIES	FAT GRAMS	CHOLES-TEROL	% OF FAT

CANDY

Item	PORTION	CAL-ORIES	FAT GRAMS	CHOLES-TEROL	% OF FAT
Almond Bar					
Plain, Nestle's	1 oz.	149	8.9	6	53.7
Golden Almond, Hershey	1.3-oz. bar	161	10.0	–	55.9
Almond Joy	1.76-oz. bar	250	14.0	–	50.4
Almonds					
Chocolate-coated	1 oz.	161	12.4	0	69.3
Sugar-coated	1 oz.	129	5.3	0	36.9
Baby Ruth	1.8-oz. bar	145	6.1	0	37.9
Bar None	1½ oz.	240	14.0	10	52.5
■Bit-o-Honey	1.7 oz. bar	200	4.0	–	16.0
■Blow Pops, Charms Junior	1	50	0.0	–	0.0
Bridge mix	1 oz.	142	6.1	–	38.7
Butterfinger	1.6-oz. bar	138	6.3	0	41.1
■Butterscotch discs	1 oz.	113	1.0	3	7.9
■Candied fruit, citron, chopped	1 oz.	89	0.1	0	1.0
■Candy corn, Brach's	1 oz.	100	0.0	0	0.0
■Candy, hard	1 oz.	109	0.0	0	0.0
Caramel					
Chocolate-coated	1 oz.	130	6.5	1	45.0
With nuts	1 oz.	121	4.6	1	34.2
Caramello	1.6 oz. bar	220	11.0	10	45.0
■Caramel roll	1 oz.	112	2.3	0	18.5
Chocolate, Cooking					
Bittersweet	1 oz.	135	11.3	0	75.3
Semisweet	1 oz.	144	10.1	0	63.1
Sweet	1 oz.	150	9.9	0	59.4
Chocolate bar, plain					
Hershey	1 oz.	153	8.8	7	51.8
Nestle's	1 oz.	149	7.9	6	47.7

■ Contains less than 20% fat   29

Item	PORTION	CAL-ORIES	FAT GRAMS	CHOLES-TEROL	% OF FAT
Chocolate bar w/nuts					
W/almonds, Cadbury	1 oz.	153	8.9	–	52.3
Hershey	1 oz.	159	10.0	8	56.6
Chocolate creams					
Vanilla	1 oz.	123	4.8	1	35.1
Coconut	1 oz.	124	5.0	0	36.3
■Dots	2¼ oz.	220	0.0	0	0.0
5th Avenue	2.1-oz. bar	290	13.0	5	40.3
Fudge					
Chocolate	1 oz.	113	3.4	0	27.0
Chocolate w/nuts	1 oz.	128	5.9	1	41.4
Vanilla	1 oz.	113	3.1	1	24.6
Vanilla, w/nuts	1 oz.	120	4.6	1	34.5
Fudge, chocolate-covered					
Without nuts	1 oz.	122	4.5	–	33.2
W/peanuts	1 oz.	128	5.9	1	41.5
Fun Fruit, Sunkist	.9 oz.	100	1.4	0	12.6
Goobers	1 oz.	160	10.0	–	56.2
■Good and Plenty	1 oz.	104	0.0	0	0.0
■Gum, Doublemint, Wrigleys	3 sticks	10	0.0	0	0.0
■Gumdrops	1 oz.	98	0.2	0	1.8
■Gummy Bears, Estee	1 piece	7	0.0	0	0.0
Halvah	1 oz.	150	10.0	–	60.0
Heathbar	1 oz.	195	9.8	–	45.2
■Jelly beans	1 oz.	104	0.1	0	0.8
■Jujyfruits	1 pc.	9	0.0	0	0.0
Kisses, Hershey	1 oz.	153	8.7	7	51.2
Kit Kat, Hershey	1 oz.	154	7.5	6	43.8
Krackel, Hershey	1 oz.	149	8.1	–	48.9
Kudos, peanut butter	1 oz.	147	9.3	–	57.0
■Licorice stick	1 oz.	99	0.4	0	3.6
■Lifesavers	1 oz.	111	0.3	0	2.4
Lollipop, Life Savers	1 piece	45	0.0	0	0.0
M & M's					
Peanut	1 oz.	143	7.1	–	44.7

■ Contains less than 20% fat

Item	PORTION	CAL-ORIES	FAT GRAMS	CHOLES-TEROL	% OF FAT
Plain	1 oz.	143	6.0	–	37.8
Malted-Milk balls	1 oz.	142	6.1	5	38.6
Mars Bar	1.8-oz. bar	240	11.0	–	41.2
■Marshmallows, large	1 oz.	90	0.0	0	0.0
■Milk Duds	1	13	0.4	–	30.8
Milky Way	2.15 oz.	280	10.0	–	32.0
Milky Way II	2.05 oz.	190	8.0	5	22.0
Mints					
■ Hard	1 oz.	103	0.6	0	5.2
Chocolate-covered	1 oz.	116	3.1	–	24.0
Mounds	1 oz.	137	7.4	0	48.6
Mr. Goodbar, Hershey	1 oz.	166	10.9	9	59.1
■Necco Wafers	2-oz. piece	228	0.0	–	0.0
Nestle's Crunch	1 oz.	149	7.9	6	47.7
Nougat/caramel, chocolate-covered	1 oz.	118	3.9	1	29.7
Oh Henry	1 oz.	140	7.0	–	45.0
$100,000 Bar	1½ oz.	200	8.0	3	36.0
Peanuts, chocolate-coated	1 oz.	159	11.7	0	66.2
Peanut bar	1 oz.	146	9.1	0	56.0
Peanut brittle	1 oz.	119	2.9	0	21.9
Peanut butter cup, Reese's	1 oz.	156	9.3	4	53.6
Peppermint Patties	1 oz.	120	3.2	–	24.0
Pom Poms	1 oz.	100	3.0	–	27.0
■Popcorn, popped, sugar-coated	1 oz.	109	1.0	0	8.3
Raisins, chocolate-coated	1 oz.	120	4.8	3	36.0
Skor Bar	1.4 oz.	220	14.0	25	57.3
Sky Bar	1½ oz.	198	7.2	–	32.7
Snickers	2-oz. bar	135	6.5	–	43.3
■Sugar Babies	1 oz.	111	1.2	–	9.7

■ Contains less than 20% fat

Item	PORTION	CAL-ORIES	FAT GRAMS	CHOLES-TEROL	% OF FAT
Three Musketeers	2.28-oz. bar	260	8.0	–	27.7
Tiger Milk, Nutri Bar, Plus Products	1 oz.	135	7.1	–	47.3
■Tootsie Roll	1 oz.	112	2.3	0	18.4
Twix	1.71-oz. bar	152	8.2	–	48.5

COOKIES

Item	PORTION	CAL-ORIES	FAT GRAMS	CHOLES-TEROL	% OF FAT
■Almond toast, Stella D'oro	1	60	1.0	0	15.0
Amaranth, Health Valley, jumbo	1	90	3.0	0	27.0
Angel bar, Stella D'oro	1	80	5.0	0	56.2
Anginetti, Stella D'oro	1	30	1.0	0	30.0
Apple Pastry, Stella D'oro	1	90	4.0	–	40.0
Animal Crackers					
Barnum	11	130	4.0	5	28.0
FFV	1	14	0.4	0	25.7
Gerber	1 piece	30	1.0	–	30.0
Nabisco	1 pkg.	255	7.8	–	27.5
■Anisette Sponge, Stella D'oro	1 piece	50	1.0	0	18.0
■Anisette Toast, Stella D'oro					
Regular	1	50	1.0	0	18.0
Jumbo	1	110	1.0	0	8.2
Apple N'Raisin, Archway	1	120	3.0	10	22.5
Apple Oatmeal Tart, Wholesome Choice, Pepperidge Farm	1	70	2.0	–	25.0

Item	PORTION	CAL-ORIES	FAT GRAMS	CHOLES-TEROL	% OF FAT
■Apple Spice, Health Valley	1	75	0.5	–	6.0
Apricot-Raspberry, Pepperidge Farm	1	50	2.0	5	36.0
Arrowroot, adult, Nabisco	1	21	0.7	–	30.0
Bordeau, Pepperidge Farm	1	35	1.5	0	38.6
Breakfast Treats, Stella D'oro	1	100	4.0	0	36.0
Brownie, w/o nuts					
Regular	1	243	10.1	10	37.4
Large, Hostess	1	243	9.6	17	35.5
Weight Watchers	1.25 oz.	100	3.0	5	27.0
Brownie w/nuts					
Regular	1	263	16.4	81	56.1
Fudge 'N Nut, Almost Home	1.2 oz.	160	7.0	–	39.4
Brussels, Pepperidge Farm					
Regular	1	55	2.5	0	40.9
Mint	1	65	3.5	0	34.6
Cameo sandwich cream, Nabisco	1	70	3.0	0	38.6
Cappuccino, Pepperidge Farm	1	50	3.0	3	54.0
Capri, Pepperidge Farm	1	80	5.0	0	56.2
Caramel Patties, FFV	1	75	3.5	–	42.0
■Carrot Walnut, Wholesome Choice, Pepperidge Farm	1	60	1.0	0	15.0
Castelets, Stella D'oro	1	70	3.0	0	38.6
Chessmen, Pepperidge Farm	1	45	2.0	5	40.0

Item	PORTION	CAL-ORIES	FAT GRAMS	CHOLES-TEROL	% OF FAT
Chiparoos, Sunshine	1	60	3.0	–	45.0
Chips Ahoy, Nabisco	1	50	2.0	–	36.0
Chocolate	1	72	3.4	13	42.5
Chocolate biscuits, Almondina	1	35	1.0	0	25.0
Chocolate chip					
Homemade	1	69	4.6	7	60.0
Estee	1	30	1.0	0	30.0
Frookie	1	45	2.0	–	40.0
Pepperidge Farm	1	50	2.7	–	48.6
Regular	1	52	2.9	5	50.2
Rich's	1	129	5.6	4	39.1
■ Snackwell's	1	10	0.2	0	1.8
Coconut					
Estee	1	30	1.0	0	30.0
Stella D'oro	1	50	2.0	–	36.0
Coconut fudge, FFV	1	80	4.0	–	45.0
Como Delight, Stella D'oro	1	150	7.0	1	42.0
■Devil's Food Cookie Cakes, Snackwell's	1	60	1.0	0	15.0
Dinosaurs, FFV	1 oz.	130	5.0	0	34.6
Dutch Cocoa, Archway	1	110	4.0	5	32.7
Fig bar, Keebler	1	65	1.5	–	20.8
■Fig Newton	1	60	1.0	–	15.0
■Fig Newtons, fat-free	1	70	0.0	0	0.0
■Fruit Bar, fat-free, Health Valley	1 bar	140	0.5	0	2.9
■Fruit Centers, fat-free, Health Valley	1	23	0.2	–	7.8
■Fruit & honey, Entenmann's	1	40	0.0	0	0.0
Fruit slices, Stella D'oro	1	60	2.0	0	30.0

■ Contains less than 20% fat   34

Item	PORTION	CAL-ORIES	FAT GRAMS	CHOLES-TEROL	% OF FAT
Fudge					
Estee	1	30	1.0	0	30.0
Stella D'oro					
Deep Night	1	65	4.0	0	55.4
Swiss	1	70	3.0	0	38.6
Geneva, Pepperidge Farm	1	65	3.0	0	41.5
Ginger Boys, FFV	1 oz.	120	4.0	0	30.0
Gingerman, Pepper-idge Farm	1	35	1.5	2	38.6
Gingersnap, small	1	36	1.3	3	32.5
■Graham Crackers, regular Sunshine	1	60	1.0	0	15.0
Graham Crackers, oat bran, Health Valley	1	14	0.4	0	25.7
■Graham Snacks, cin-namon, Snackwell's	9	50	0.0	0	0.0
Granola bar, chocolate chip					
Quaker	1 oz.	129	5.0	–	34.9
New Trail	1.3-oz. bar	142	6.8	–	43.1
Granola bar, dipped, caramel nut, Quaker	1.1-oz. bar	131	5.6	–	38.5
Granola bar, honey & oats					
Health Valley	1 oz.	105	4.0	–	34.3
Quaker	1 oz.	129	5.0	–	34.8
Granola Bar, peanut butter/chocolate chip, Quaker	1 oz.	131	5.5	–	37.8
■Health Valley, fat-free, cholester-ol-free	3	75	0.0	0	0.0
Hydrox, Sunshine	1	50	2.0	0	36.0
Ice Cream Cone					
■ Sugar, Keebler	1	45	0.0	0	0.0

■ Contains less than 20% fat

Item	PORTION	CAL-ORIES	FAT GRAMS	CHOLES-TEROL	% OF FAT
■ Waffle cone, Keebler	1	100	1.0	0	9.0
Lemon Nut, X-Large, Pepperidge Farm	1	337	17.9	–	47.8
Lido, Pepperidge Farm	1	90	5.0	1	50.0
■Jammers	1	41	0.4	0	9.0
Linzer, Pepperidge Farm	1	120	4.0	3	30.0
Love, Stella D'oro	1	110	5.0	0	40.9
Macaroons	1	59	2.3	0	35.1
Mallopuffs, Sunshine	1	70	2.0	–	25.0
Milano, Pepperidge Farm	1	75	3.5	2	42.0
Molasses, big, Grand-ma's	1	160	4.5	2	25.3
* Oatmeal, homemade	1	37	1.0	0	24.0
Oatmeal, plain	1	57	2.7	9	42.6
Oatmeal/raisin, regu-lar	1	63	2.7	8	38.6
Archway	1	100	3.0	–	27.0
■ Fat-free, Entenmann's	1	80	0.0	0	0.0
■ Fat-free, R. W. Frookie	1	50	0.2	–	3.0
Pepperidge Farm	1	57	2.7	–	42.6
Oreo	1	51	1.5	–	26.5
Double Stuf, Nabisco	1	70	4.0	2	51.4
Orleans, Pepperidge Farm	1	30	2.0	–	60.0
Peach-Apricot Bar, vanilla, FFV	1	70	1.0	0	12.9
Peanut butter, home-made	1	102	6.0	11	53.9

■ Contains less than 20% fat   36   * See page xxxii

Item	PORTION	CAL-ORIES	FAT GRAMS	CHOLES-TEROL	% OF FAT
Peanut butter fudge, Almost Home	1	140	7.0	–	45.0
Pfeffernusse, Stella D'oro	1	40	1.0	0	22.5
Pirouette, Pepperidge Farm	1	35	2.0	–	51.4
Praline Pecan, FFV	1	40	2.0	–	45.0
Prune pastry, Stella D'oro	1	90	4.0	–	40.0
Raisin, soft, big, Grandma's	1	160	5.0	5	28.1
■Raspberry Tart, Wholesome Choice, Pepperidge Farm	1	60	1.0	–	15.0
Rice Krispie Square	1	226	6.2	1	24.7
Rocky Road, Archway	1	130	6.0	10	41.5
Royal Dainty, FFV	1	60	3.0	–	45.0
■Royal Nuggets, Stella D'oro	1	2	0.0	–	0.0
Sandwich, Chocolate Chocolate-covered	4	180	8.0	0	40.0
Cream filled, Grandma's	1	260	12.0	0	41.5
Shortbread, Lorna Doone	1	36	2.0	–	50.0
Social Tea, Nabisco	1	22	0.7	–	28.6
Strawberry, Pepperidge Farm	1	50	2.5	5	45.0
Strawberry filled, Archway	1	100	3.0	10	27.0
Sugar, soft, thick	1	31	1.2	0	34.8
Sugar wafer	1	47	2.4	7	45.9
Sweet Spots, Keebler	1	25	1.5	–	54.0
Tahiti, Pepperidge Farm	1	90	6.0	5	60.0

■ Contains less than 20% fat

Item	PORTION	CAL-ORIES	FAT GRAMS	CHOLES-TEROL	% OF FAT
Tango, FFV	1	80	2.5	–	28.1
Toy, Sunshine	1	12	0.4	0	30.0
Vanilla creme, French, Keebler	1	83	3.6	–	39.0
■Vanilla Rocky Road, B. P. Gourmet	1	18	0.0	0	0.0
Vanilla wafer					
Homemade	1	17	0.9	2	47.6
Nilla Wafers	1	13	0.4	–	27.7

CRACKERS

Item	PORTION	CAL-ORIES	FAT GRAMS	CHOLES-TEROL	% OF FAT
Al-Mak Original Sesame	1 oz.	45	2.0	–	40.0
Bacon flavor thins, Nabisco	1	10	0.6	0	54.0
Butter thin, Pepperidge Farm	1	17	0.7	–	37.1
Cheese Nips	1 oz.	132	5.7	–	38.9
Cheese & peanut butter, Nabisco	1 oz.	132	5.7	–	38.9
Cheese Wheels, Health Valley	1 oz.	140	9.0	–	57.8
Cheez-It, Sunshine	½ oz.	140	8.0	4	51.4
Chic in Biskit	½ oz.	160	10.0	0	56.2
■Cinnamon Treat, Nabisco	1	30	0.5	–	15.0
Club, Keebler	1	15	0.7	–	42.0
Crown Pilot, Nabisco	1	70	2.0	0	25.7
■English Water Biscuit, Pepperidge Farm	1	17	0.2	0	10.6
Escort, Nabisco	1	23	1.3	0	50.9
Fiber Rich Bran	2	35	0.8	0	20.6
■Finn Crisp	1	38	0.0	0	0.0
Goldfish, Pepperidge Farm					
Cheese	1 oz.	140	6.8	–	43.7

■ Contains less than 20% fat   38

Item	PORTION	CAL-ORIES	FAT GRAMS	CHOLES-TEROL	% OF FAT
Parmesan	1 oz.	120	4.0	0	30.0
Pizza	1 oz.	130	5.0	–	34.6
Pretzel	1 oz.	116	2.6	–	20.1
Hi Ho	½ oz.	160	10.0	0	56.2
■Kavli	1 oz.	99	0.7	0	6.4
■Matzo, plain	1 oz.	109	0.5	0	4.1
■Matzo w/bran, Whole wheat	1 oz.	110	0.8	0	6.5
Meal Mates, Nabisco	1	23	1.0	0	39.1
Melba Toast,					
■ Plain	1 oz.	122	1.0	0	7.0
Sesame rounds, Keebler	1 oz.	119	3.4	–	25.7
Oyster cracker					
Keebler, Large	1 oz.	125	3.7	–	26.6
■ Nabisco	½ oz.	120	2.0	0	15.0
Peanut Butter and Cheese	1 oz.	168	12.1	1	64.8
■Premium, no fat, Nabisco	½ oz.	100	0.0	0	0.0
■Rice cake, plain, un-salted, Chico San	1 oz.	110	0.8	0	6.5
■Rice Hol-Grain	1	112	0.5	0	4.0
Ritz, Nabisco	1 oz.	150	8.6	0	51.6
Ritz Bits, Nabisco	1 oz.	140	8.0	0	51.4
Royal Lunch	1	60	2.0	–	30.0
■Rye	1 oz.	106	0.0	0	0.0
■Rye, crisp bread, Wasa	1 oz.	100	0.0	0	0.0
Ry krisp					
■ Original	1 oz.	102	0.2	0	1.8
■ Seasoned	1 oz.	110	2.0	0	16.4
■Saltine	1 oz.	129	2.6	–	18.1
Schooners, FFV					
Regular	½ oz.	60	2.0	0	30.0
Whole wheat	½ oz.	70	4.0	0	51.4

■ Contains less than 20% fat   39

Item	PORTION	CAL-ORIES	FAT GRAMS	CHOLES-TEROL	% OF FAT
Sociables	1 oz.	153	6.5	–	38.2
Soda	1 oz.	124	3.7	0	26.8
Tams, Manischewitz	10 pieces	147	8.0	–	49.0
Triscuit	1 oz.	142	4.7	0	29.8
Uneeda Biscuit, Nabisco	3	90	3.0	0	30.0
Vegetable Thins, Nabisco	7	70	4.4	0	56.6
Waverly Wafer	1 oz.	131	3.7	–	25.4
■Wheat, fat-free, Health Valley	½ g.	40	.5	–	11.3
Wheat, sesame, Pepperidge Farm	1 oz.	123	6.2	0	45.4
■ Snackwell's, Nabisco	5	50	1.0	–	18.0
■ Wasa Crispbread	0.5 oz.	50	0.0	0	0.0
Wheatsworth	1 oz.	140	6.0	0	38.6
Wheat Thins					
Nutty	1 oz.	140	8.0	0	51.4
Regular	1 oz.	142	6.0	0	38.0
Whole wheat	1 oz.	132	5.3	0	36.1
■Manischewitz	1	9	0.1	–	10.0
■ Organic, Health Valley, fat free	0.5 oz.	40	0.0	0	0.0
■Zwieback	1 oz.	120	2.5	3	18.7

DAIRY & DAIRY PRODUCTS

Cheese

Item	PORTION	CAL-ORIES	FAT GRAMS	CHOLES-TEROL	% OF FAT
■Alpine Lace, Free n' Lean	1 oz.	40	0.0	5	0.0
Alpine Lace	1 oz.	90	6.0	20	90.0
■American, Kraft Free	1 oz.	45	0.0	5	0.0
Light 'N' Lively	1 oz.	69	4.0	15	52.2
American, pasturized					
Churny Lite	1 oz.	80	5.0	20	56.2
Dorman's Lo-chol	1 oz.	90	0.0	–	–

Item	PORTION	CAL-ORIES	FAT GRAMS	CHOLES-TEROL	% OF FAT
Lite Line	1 oz.	50	2.0	–	36.0
Blue	1 oz.	100	8.1	21	72.9
Brick, Land O' Lakes	1 oz.	110	8.0	25	65.4
Brie	1 oz.	95	7.8	28	73.9
Camembert	1 oz.	85	6.9	20	73.1
Caraway	1 oz.	107	8.3	24	69.8
Cheddar, regular					
Land O' Lakes	1 oz.	110	9.0	30	73.6
Lucerne, mellow or sharp	1 oz.	110	10.0	30	81.8
■ Lifetime, non-fat	1 oz.	40	0.0	3	0.0
Cheddar, low-fat					
Cheddar Delite, Dorman Lite	1 oz.	80	5.0	–	56.2
Lifetime	1 oz.	64	3.0	9	42.2
Pasturized, Light 'N' Lively	1 oz.	69	4.0	15	52.2
Cheezbits, processed Gruyere	1 cube	8	0.4	–	45.0
Colby					
Alpine Lace Lo	1 oz.	80	5.0	20	56.2
Churny Lite	1 oz.	80	5.0	20	56.2
Dorman's Lo-Chol	1 oz.	100	7.0	3	63.0
Land O' Lakes	1 oz.	110	9.0	25	73.6
Cottage, creamed, small curd	½ cup	108	4.7	16	39.2
Cottage, low-fat					
■ 1% fat	½ cup	81	1.1	5	12.2
■ 2% fat	½ cup	102	2.2	9	19.4
Cottage, non-fat					
Knudsen	½ cup	70	0.0	5	0.0
■ Light 'N' Lively	½ cup	90	0.0	10	0.0
Cream, regular, Philadelphia	1 oz.	98	9.6	28	88.2
■Cream, Imitation Weight Watchers	1 oz.	22	0.4	1	16.4

■ Contains less than 20% fat   41

Item	PORTION	CAL-ORIES	FAT GRAMS	CHOLES-TEROL	% OF FAT
Cream, light					
Lite, Neufchatel, Kraft	1 oz.	74	6.6	22	80.2
Light, reduced fat, Philadelphia	1 oz.	60	5.0	10	75.0
■Cream, non-fat, Free, Philadelphia	1 oz.	25	0.0	5	0.0
Edam, Churny May-Bud	1 oz.	100	8.0	25	72.0
Farmer's, Friendship, regular or un-salted	1 oz.	40	3.0	10	67.5
Feta, natural, Churny	1 oz.	75	6.5	25	78.0
Fondue, homemade	1 oz.	75	5.2	64	62.4
Gouda, Churny May-Bud					
Regular	1 oz.	100	8.0	–	72.0
Lite	1 oz.	81	5.0	15	55.6
Hoop, natural, Friendship, no salt added	1 oz.	21	0.5	2	21.4
Jack, Land O' Lakes	1 oz.	90	8.0	20	80.0
Jarlsberg, Lite, Naseland Farms	1 oz.	80	4.0	15	45.0
Jarlsberg, Norwegian, Safeway	1 oz.	100	8.0	24	72.0
Limburger	1 oz.	93	7.7	26	74.5
Longhorn, Safeway	1 oz.	110	10.0	30	81.8
Monterey Jack					
Alpine Lace Monti-Jack-Lo	1 oz.	80	5.0	15	56.2
Kraft	1 oz.	105	8.6	29	73.7
Lifetime	1 oz.	64	3.0	9	42.2
Weight Watchers	1 oz.	80	5.0	15	56.2
Mozzarella					
Light					
■ Alpine Lace, Free 'n' Lean	1 oz.	40	0.0	5	0.0

■ Contains less than 20% fat

Item	PORTION	CALORIES	FAT GRAMS	CHOLESTEROL	% OF FAT
Dorman's	1 oz.	80	4.0	17	45.0
■ Polly-O-Free	1 oz.	40	0.0	5	0.0
Low cholesterol					
Dorman's	1 oz.	90	6.0	3	60.0
Lifetime	1 oz.	60	2.0	7	30.0
Low moisture, Casino	1 oz.	90	7.0	25	70.0
Part skim milk					
Low moisture	1 oz.	79	4.9	15	55.8
Alpine Lace	1 oz.	70	5.0	15	64.3
Frigo, reduced fat	1 oz.	60	3.0	10	45.0
Kraft	1 oz.	79	5.2	17	59.2
Polly-O, regular	1 oz.	80	5.0	15	56.2
Smoked	1 oz.	85	7.0	25	74.1
Whole milk, Polly-O					
Regular	1 oz.	90	6.0	20	60.0
Fior di Latte	1 oz.	80	6.0	20	67.5
Muenster					
Alpine Lace	1 oz.	100	8.0	30	72.0
Land O' Lakes	1 oz.	100	9.0	25	81.0
Lifetime	1 oz.	70	5.0	–	64.3
Neufchatel	1 oz.	74	6.6	22	80.2
Old English, pasturized, Kraft	1 oz.	105	8.7	27	74.6
Parmesan, grated	1 oz.	129	8.5	22	59.3
Kraft	1 oz.	128	8.6	29	60.5
Sargento, Preferred Light	1 oz.	40	2.0	10	45.0
Port Du Salut	1 oz.	100	8.0	35	72.0
Processed					
■ Alpine Lace Free 'N Lean	1 oz.	40	0.0	–	0.0
American, cold pack	1 oz.	94	6.9	18	66.1
American, pasturized	1 oz.	93	7.0	18	67.7

■ Contains less than 20% fat

Item	PORTION	CAL-ORIES	FAT GRAMS	CHOLES-TEROL	% OF FAT
Extra Sharp, Cracker Barrel	1 oz.	93	6.8	19	65.8
Hot Pepper, Land O' Lakes	1 oz.	93	6.9	18	66.7
■ Kraft Free, singles	1 oz.	45	0.0	–	0.0
Kraft Light, singles	1 oz.	70	4.0	15	70.0
Pimiento, Land O' Lakes	1 oz.	107	9.0	23	75.7
Smoked Flavor, Weight Watchers	1 oz.	71	4.1	–	51.9
Swiss	1 oz.	95	7.1	24	67.3
Velveeta, Kraft	1 oz.	83	6.0	19	65.1
Velveeta Light, Kraft singles	1 oz.	70	4.0	–	51.4
Weight Watchers	1 oz.	50	2.0	–	36.0
Provolone					
Alpine Lace Provo-Lo	1 oz.	70	5.0	15	64.3
Dorman's light	1 oz.	80	4.0	17	45.0
Lucerne, sliced	1 oz.	100	8.0	20	72.0
■ Quark, non-fat, Apple Farms	½ cup	71	0.0	65	0.0
Ricotta					
■ Fat free, Polly-O	½ cup	100	0.0	5	0.0
Light					
Polly-O	1 oz.	40	2.0	5	45.0
Sargento, Lite	½ cup	75	3.2	12	30.3
Truly Lite, Frigo	1 oz.	30	1.0	7	30.0
Part skim milk, Polly-O	1 oz.	45	3.0	10	60.0
Whole milk, Polly-O	1 oz.	50	3.5	17	63.0
Romano, grated, Progresso	1 tb.	23	2.0	6	78.3
Roquefort	1 oz.	105	8.7	26	74.6

Item	PORTION	CAL- ORIES	FAT GRAMS	CHOLES- TEROL	% OF FAT
Slim Jack, Lite, Dorman	1 oz.	80	5.0	18	56.2
■Smart Beat, Nucoa, imitation cheese slices, all vari- eties	1 oz.	45	0.0	0	0.0
Spread					
American, pasturized	1 oz.	82	6.0	16	65.8
Cheese Whiz, Kraft	1 oz.	77	5.8	18	67.8
Port Wine, Weight Watchers	2 tb.	40	2.0	10	45.0
Substitute or Imitation					
American					
Formägg slices	1 oz.	93	7.0	–	67.7
Soyco singles	1 oz.	80	5.0	–	56.2
Weight Watchers slices	1 oz.	50	2.0	5	36.0
Cheddar					
Frigo	1 oz.	90	7.0	0	57.0
Soya Kaas	1 oz.	79	5.0	–	57.0
Weight Watchers slices	1 oz.	50	2.0	5	36.0
Nucoa Heart Beat	1 oz.	50	2.0	0	36.0
NûTofû	1 oz.	85	6.0	–	67.5
■ Soya Melt, White Wave, fat-free	1 oz.	40	0.0	–	0.0
Swiss, regular, Lu- cerne	1 oz.	100	8.0	24	72.0
Swiss, light					
Alpine Lace Swiss-Lo	1 oz.	100	7.0	20	63.0
Churny Lite	1 oz.	90	5.0	20	50.0
Kraft Light Natu- rals	1 oz.	90	5.0	20	50.0
■ Lifetime, non-fat	1 oz.	40	0.0	3	0.0

Item	PORTION	CAL-ORIES	FAT GRAMS	CHOLES-TEROL	% OF FAT
Sargento, Preferred Light	1 oz.	80	4.0	15	45.0
Weight Watchers, skim, semisoft	1 oz.	80	5.2	–	58.5
Swiss slices, Weight Watchers	1 oz.	50	2.0	15	36.0
Swiss, no salt, Dorman's	1 oz.	100	8.0	25	72.0

Milk & Milk Beverages
■Alba 77, dry

Item	PORTION	CAL-ORIES	FAT GRAMS	CHOLES-TEROL	% OF FAT
Chocolate	1 pkt.	70	1.0	–	12.9
Vanilla	1 pkt.	70	0.0	0	0.0
■Buttermilk, whole	1 cup	98	2.1	10	19.3
■Buttermilk, low fat	1 cup	120	4.0	14	30.0
■Buttermilk, dried	¼ cup	465	7.0	83	14.0
■ Poland, prepared	1 cup	79	0.7	5	8.0
Cocoa beverage, w/whole milk	1 cup	217	10.2	2	42.3
Cocoa mix, regular, Swiss Miss	1 env.	110	3.0	0	24.5

■Cocoa mix, low calorie Swiss Miss

Item	PORTION	CAL-ORIES	FAT GRAMS	CHOLES-TEROL	% OF FAT
Regular	1 env.	70	0.8	–	10.3
W/sugar-free mini marsh-mallows	1 env.	50	0.5	0	9.0
Weight Watchers	1 env.	60	0.0	–	0.0

Coffee creamers, dairy and non-dairy

Item	PORTION	CAL-ORIES	FAT GRAMS	CHOLES-TEROL	% OF FAT
Coffee-Mate, liquid, non-dairy	1 tb.	10	0.8	0	72.0

Coffee-Mate powder

Item	PORTION	CAL-ORIES	FAT GRAMS	CHOLES-TEROL	% OF FAT
Regular	1 tsp.	10	0.5	0	45.0
Lite	1 tsp.	8	0.4	0	45.0
Coffee-Rich, frozen liquid	1 tb.	22	1.6	0	65.4

Item	PORTION	CAL-ORIES	FAT GRAMS	CHOLES-TEROL	% OF FAT
Cremora	1 tsp.	12	1.0	–	75.0
Mocha mix, light	1 tb.	20	2.0	0	90.0
■ Weight Watchers dairy creamer	1 env.	10	0.1	–	9.0
Condensed, sweet-ened, canned, Carnation	2 tb.	123	3.3	9	24.1
Cream, half & half, Johanna Farms	1 tb.	20	1.7	6	76.5
Cream, heavy whip-ping, Land O' Lakes	1 tb.	50	5.0	15	90.0
Cream, light, (coffee or table)	1 tb.	29	2.9	10	90.0
Cream, light, (whipping)					
Whipped	2 tb.	44	4.6	17	94.1
Unwhipped	2 tb.	87	9.2	33	95.2
Cream, sour	2 tb.	62	6.0	13	87.1
Half and Half,	2 tb.	41	3.6	11	79.0
Cream, sour, light					
■ Knudsen, fat free	2 tb.	18	0.0	0	0.0
Land O' Lakes w/chives	2 tb.	40	2.0	4	45.0
■ Light 'N' Lively Free	2 tb.	16	0.0	0	0.0
Weight Watchers	2 tb.	34	2.0	–	52.9
Cream, sour, imita-tion, Pet	2 tb.	50	4.0	0	72.0
■Eggnog, light, Borden	1 cup	130	2.0	80	14.0
Eggnog, non-alcoholic, Johanna	1 cup	391	15.2	149	35.0
Evaporated milk, whole, Lucerne	1 cup	170	20.0	–	52.9
Evaporated milk, low fat, Carnation	1 cup	216	4.8	35	20.0

■ Contains less than 20% fat   47

Item	PORTION	CAL-ORIES	FAT GRAMS	CHOLES-TEROL	% OF FAT
■Evaporated milk, skim, Pet 99	1 cup	200	0.0	2	0.0
■Lactaid	1 cup	90	0.0	0	0.0
Milk, dry					
■ Non-fat, instant, Lucerne	1 cup	80	1.0	–	11.2
Whole	¼ cup	159	8.5	31	48.1
Milk, chocolate					
Low fat					
■ 1% fat	1 cup	158	2.5	8	14.2
2% fat	1 cup	180	5.0	18	25.0
Hershey's, 2% fat	1 cup	190	5.0	20	23.7
■ Land O' Lakes, ½% fat	1 cup	150	1.0	5	6.0
Whole					
Hershey's	1 cup	210	9.0	–	38.6
Johanna	1 cup	200	8.0	30	36.0
Nestlé Quik	1 cup	220	8.0	–	32.7
■Milk, acidophilus, Borden, 1% fat	1 cup	110	2.0	10	16.0
Milk, goat	1 cup	168	9.8	27	52.5
Milk, low fat, Lucerne					
◪ ½, 1, or 1½% fat	1 cup	90	1.0	–	10.0
2% fat	1 cup	120	5.0	–	37.5
Milk, non-fat					
■ Johanna	1 cup	80	0.0	4	0.0
■ Knudsen	1 cup	80	0.0	–	0.0
■Milk, skim					
Land O' Lakes	1 cup	90	1.0	5	10.0
Weight Watchers	1 cup	90	0.5	–	5.0
Milk, whole					
3.3% fat	1 cup	149	8.1	34	48.9
Johanna	1 cup	150	8.0	33	48.0
Milk, malted, chocolate	1 cup	233	9.1	34	35.1
Natural flavor	1 cup	236	10.0	37	38.1

■ Contains less than 20% fat   48

Item	PORTION	CALORIES	FAT GRAMS	CHOLESTEROL	% OF FAT
Milkshake					
Chocolate	1 cup	282	6.4	24	20.4
Thick, frosty	1 cup	622	27.6	–	39.0
Vanilla	1 cup	265	7.1	28	24.1
■Quik, Nestle's					
Chocolate	2 tb.	36	0.5	0	12.5
Strawberry	2 tb.	41	0.0	0	0.0
■Slender, chocolate fudge, Carnation	10 oz.	220	4.0	4	16.4
Yogurt					
Regular					
Plain					
Regular, Yoplait	6 oz.	130	3.0	15	20.8
Low fat, Lucerne	1 cup	160	5.0	20	28.1
■ Non-fat, Dannon	1 cup	110	0.0	5	0.0
■ Flavored					
Coffee, Dannon	1 cup	200	3.0	10	13.5
Vanilla, Dannon Light	1 cup	100	0.0	4	0.0
Vanilla, Friendship	1 cup	210	3.0	14	12.9
■ Fruit varieties, regular					
Apple, dutch, Dannon	1 cup	240	3.0	10	11.2
Blueberry, Yoplait	6 oz.	190	3.0	10	14.2
Lemon, Johanna	1 cup	220	4.0	–	16.4
Peach, Dannon	1 cup	240	3.0	10	11.2
Pineapple, Yoplait	6 oz.	190	3.0	10	14.2
Raspberry, Dannon Fresh Flavors	1 cup	200	4.0	10	18.0
Strawberry, Yoplait	6 oz.	190	4.0	20	18.9

■ Contains less than 20% fat   49

Item	PORTION	CAL-ORIES	FAT GRAMS	CHOLES-TEROL	% OF FAT
Fruit varieties, light, Yoplait	6 oz.	90	0.0	3	0.0
Fruit varieties, low fat, Lucerne	1 cup	260	4.0	15	13.8
■ Fruit variety, non-fat					
Alta Dena, non-fat, fruit	1 cup	190	1.0	–	4.0
Colombo, non-fat, fruit	1 cup	190	1.0	5	5.0
Fruit flavors, Lite 'N' Lively	1 cup	100	0.0	5	0.0
Weight Watchers, Ultima 90	1 cup	90	0.0	5	0.0
Frozen (see Ice Cream, Frozen Yogurt & Non-dairy Frozen Desserts)					
Frozen, soft-serve, Baskin-Robbins					
■ Banana, raspberry or strawberry	4 fl. oz.	124	1.6	8	11.6
■ Coconut	4 fl. oz.	144	4.0	8	11.1
■ Mocha, Truly Free	4 fl. oz.	70	0.0	0	0.0
Peanut butter	4 fl. oz.	148	4.4	8	26.7
■ Strawberry, non-fat	4 fl. oz.	110	0.0	0	0.0

DESSERTS

Cakes

Item	PORTION	CAL-ORIES	FAT GRAMS	CHOLES-TEROL	% OF FAT
Angel Food					
■ Duncan Hines, prepared	2 oz.	233	0.0	0	0.0
■ Un-iced, Chef Fran	2 oz.	166	0.1	–	0.5
Apple, Dolly Madison	2 oz.	227	8.0	–	31.7
Apple cinnamon, prepared, Betty Crocker Supermoist					
Regular	1/12 of cake	250	10.0	55	36.0
No cholesterol recipe	1/12 of cake	210	6.0	0	25.7

■ Contains less than 20% fat

Item	PORTION	CAL-ORIES	FAT GRAMS	CHOLES-TEROL	% OF FAT
■Apple spice, Entenmann's, fat & cholesterol free	2 oz.	160	0.0	0	0.0
Banana, Sara Lee	2 oz.	200	7.8	–	35.1
■Banana crunch, Entenmann's, fat & cholesterol free	2 oz.	160	0.0	0	0.0
Black forest	2 oz.	179	6.8	61	34.2
Black forest cherry, Pillsbury Bundt	⅟16 of cake	240	8.0	–	30.0
■Blueberry crunch, Entenmann's, fat & cholesterol free	2 oz.	140	0.0	0	0.0
Butter Brickle, prepared, Betty Crocker Supermoist					
Regular	⅟12 of cake	250	10.0	55	36.0
No cholesterol	⅟12 of cake	220	6.0	0	24.5
Butter French Orient, Entenmann's	1.6 oz.	180	8.0	–	40.0
Butter Pound, Sara Lee	1 oz.	130	7.0	–	48.0
Butter streusel, Dolly Madison	2 oz.	200	8.0	–	36.0
Carrot					
Homemade	2 oz.	203	11.9	32	52.8
Pepperidge Farm	2 oz.	204	11.6	–	51.2
Pillsbury	2″ × 3″ slice	295	15.6	–	47.6
Sara Lee	2 oz.	215	12.0	–	50.2
Weight Watchers	2 oz.	108	2.7	17	22.5
Cheesecake, homemade					
Regular	2 oz.	188	13.7	64	65.6
Prepared from mix, w/crust, Jell-O	2 oz.	164	7.8	16	42.8

■ Contains less than 20% fat

Item	PORTION	CAL-ORIES	FAT GRAMS	CHOLES-TEROL	% OF FAT
* Pumpkin Cheesecake, frozen, French Cream, Sara Lee	1 serv.	129	4.5	10	31.3
French Cream, Sara Lee	2 oz.	167	10.9	–	58.7
French Strawberry Cheesecake, Sara Lee	3.7 oz.	240	13.0	20.0	49.0
■ Lights Strawberry French Cheese-cake, Sara Lee	1.23 oz.	150	2.0	5.0	12.0
■ Strawberry Cheese-cake, Weight Watchers	1 individual	180	4.0	20.0	20.0
Chocolate, homemade					
* Chocoholics	2 oz.	94	4.1	0	39.2
Chocolate, w/chocolate icing	2 oz.	174	6.4	29	33.1
Chocolate, commercial					
■ Loaf, non-fat, Entenmann's	2 oz.	140	0.0	0	0.0
Sheet, Awrey	2 oz.	210	8.4	52	36.0
Chocolate, frozen					
■ Fat free, Sara Lee	2 oz.	136	0.0	0	0.0
Chocolate fudge, layer, Pepperidge Farm	2 oz.	222	12.3	–	49.9
Cinnamon					
Dolly Madison Buttercrumb	2 oz.	227	10.7	–	42.3
Pillsbury, prepared, Streusel Swirl	⅛ of cake	240	11.0	–	41.2
Cinnamon pecan streusel, Betty Crocker MicroRave					
Regular	⅙ of cake	290	13.0	45	40.3
No cholesterol recipe	⅙ of cake	240	8.0	0	30.0

Item	PORTION	CALORIES	FAT GRAMS	CHOLESTEROL	% OF FAT
Coconut, Layer, Pepperidge Farms	2 oz.	222	11.1	–	45.0
Coffee cake					
Sara Lee, pecan	2.3 oz.	280	16.0	–	51.4
Weight Watchers	2.3 oz.	190	7.0	–	33.1
■Coffee cake, cherry filled, Entenmann's, fat & cholesterol free	2 oz.	138	0.0	0	0.0
■Cranberry Orange, Entenmann's Fat-free	1 oz.	70	0.0	0	0.0
* Cupcake, Chocolate Zucchini	2 oz.	99	2.7	1	24.5
Cupcake, homemade, w/egg/milk w/chocolate icing	2 oz.	203	7.1	27	31.5
w/white icing	2 oz.	200	6.0	0	27.0
Cupcake, commercial or frozen					
Chocolate, Hostess	2 oz.	181	5.1	6	25.4
Yellow, chocolate iced, Stouffer's	2 oz.	219	7.4	–	30.4
Devil's Food, homemade, w/chocolate icing	2 oz.	192	7.0	27	32.8
Devil's Food, prepared					
Betty Crocker	2 oz.	351	16.2	74	41.5
Pillsbury Plus w/icing, frozen	2 oz.	364	20.2	94	49.9
Ding Dongs, Hostess	2 oz.	261	15.3	10	52.8
Fruit cake, light, homemade	2 oz.	221	9.4	0	38.3

Item	PORTION	CAL-ORIES	FAT GRAMS	CHOLES-TEROL	% OF FAT
Fudge Brownie, Swiss Mocha, Weight Watchers	1.23 oz.	90	2.0	25	20.0
Fudge Cake, Double, Weight Watchers	2.75 oz.	180	4.0	5	20.0
German chocolate layer, Pepperidge Farm	2 oz.	222	12.3	–	49.8
Gingerbread, homemade					
Made with milk	2 oz.	180	6.0	1	30.0
Made with water	2 oz.	156	3.9	0	22.5
Golden Layer, Pepperidge Farm	2 oz.	222	11.1	–	45.0
■Golden Loaf, non-fat, Entenmann's	2 oz.	160	0.0	0	0.0
Ho Ho's, Hostess	2 oz.	238	11.9	–	45.0
Icing, homemade					
■ Caramel	2 oz.	77	1.4	5	16.4
■ Chocolate	2 oz.	42	0.7	0	15.0
Chocolate Fudge	2 oz.	147	5.5	8	33.7
■ Coconut	2 oz.	38	0.8	0	18.9
■ Fudge, creamy, made w/water	2 oz.	52	1.0	0	17.3
■ White, boiled	2 oz.	51	1.0	3	17.6
■ White, uncooked	2 oz.	75	1.3	4	15.6
Icing, commercial					
Chocolate Fudge, Pillsbury Supreme	2 oz.	150	6.0	0	36.0
Coconut Pecan, Pillsbury Supreme	2 oz.	160	6.0	0	33.8
Cream Cheese, Ampco	2 oz.	128	6.5	7	45.7

Item	PORTION	CALORIES	FAT GRAMS	CHOLESTEROL	% OF FAT
Lemon, w/lemon glaze	2 oz.	187	4.9	22	23.6
Lemon Creme Cake, light, Sara Lee	1 piece	180	6.0	10	60.0
Marble, w/white icing	2 oz.	188	4.9	29	23.5
*■Pineapple	2 oz.	113	1.8	0	14.3
■Pineapple, Crunch, non-fat, Entenmann's	2 oz.	140	0.0	0	0.0
Pineapple upside down	2 oz.	145	6.6	14	40.9
Pound Cake					
Homemade, w/o icing	2 oz.	234	13.4	103	51.5
Dolly Madison	2 oz.	189	6.9	–	32.7
Pepperidge Farm, no cholesterol	2 oz.	220	12.0	0	49.1
Sara Lee	2 oz.	208	9.4	–	40.7
■ Free & Light	⅒ of cake	70	0.0	0	0.0
Shortcake, strawberry, Pepperidge Farm Dessert Lights	2 oz.	113	3.3	47	26.5
Sno Ball, Hostess	2 oz.	181	5.1	3	25.3
Spice, Betty Crocker Supermoist, prepared					
Regular	1/12 of cake	260	11.0	55	38.1
No cholesterol	1/12 of cake	220	7.0	0	28.6
Sponge, homemade, w/o icing,	2 oz.	162	4.4	196	24.4
*■Tea loaf, spiced honey	2 oz.	47	0.9	0	17.2
Twinkie, regular, Hostess	2 oz.	193	5.7	28	26.6

Item	PORTION	CAL-ORIES	FAT GRAMS	CHOLES-TEROL	% OF FAT
Vanilla					
Betty Crocker MicroRave, with frosting	⅙ of cake	320	17.0	35	47.8
Pepperidge Farm, layer	1.7 oz.	190	8.0	20	37.9
White, w/chocolate icing	2 oz.	180	6.6	1	33.0
Yellow, w/chocolate icing	2 oz.	175	6.2	29	31.9
Pies					
Apple					
Homemade	3 oz.	179	6.7	5	33.7
Banquet, family size	3 oz.	225	9.9	–	39.6
Mrs. Smith's					
Regular	3¼ oz.	220	10.0	0	40.9
Natural Juice	4.6 oz.	370	20.0	0	48.6
Pie In Minutes	3.1 oz.	210	9.0	0	38.6
Weight Watchers	3½ oz.	200	5.0	5	22.5
Banana cream	3 oz.	166	6.7	57	36.0
Banquet	3 oz.	232	12.9	–	49.9
Pet-Ritz	3 oz.	222	11.7	–	47.6
Banana, custard	3 oz.	138	6.0	77	39.1
Blackberry	3 oz.	163	5.3	2	29.3
Blueberry	3 oz.	157	5.4	2	30.9
Banquet	3.3 oz.	270	11.0	–	36.7
Dolly Madison	4.5 oz.	430	21.0	–	43.9
Mrs. Smith's Pie In Minutes	3.1 oz.	220	9.0	0	36.8
Boston cream	3 oz.	175	6.0	57	30.9
Cherry	3 oz.	149	5.4	0	32.6
Mrs. Smith's Natural Juice	3 oz.	228	10.4	0	41.2
Pet-Ritz	3 oz.	209	8.4	–	36.0
Chocolate cream	3 oz.	180	7.7	63	38.5

■ Contains less than 20% fat   56

Item	PORTION	CAL-ORIES	FAT GRAMS	CHOLES-TEROL	%-OF FAT
Chocolate meringue	3 oz.	180	6.8	55	34.0
Chocolate mocha, Weight Watchers	1	160	5.0	5	28.1
Coconut cream	3 oz.	196	9.8	61	45.0
Coconut custard	3 oz.	171	9.8	82	51.6
■Key lime, gelatine base	3 oz.	100	1.7	7	15.3
Lemon chiffon	3 oz.	232	11.9	110	46.2
Lemon cream, Mrs. Smith's	3 oz.	242	11.9	4	43.1
Lemon meringue	3 oz.	189	4.9	26	23.3
Mincemeat, Chef Pierre	3 oz.	242	10.5	9	39.0
Mississippi Mud, Pepperidge Farm	3 oz.	413	30.7	80	66.8
Neapolitan, Pet-Ritz	3 oz.	232	12.9	–	49.9
Peach snack, Hostess	3 oz.	266	14.6	20	49.4
Peach, Chef Pierre, individual	3 oz.	202	8.2	8	36.5
Pecan	3 oz.	310	13.2	92	38.3
Pumpkin	3 oz.	136	5.1	46	33.7
Raisin	3 oz.	316	9.9	3	28.2
Rhubarb	3 oz.	190	5.9	3	27.9
Strawberry	3 oz.	144	5.1	0	31.8
Sweet potato	3 oz.	151	5.2	47	31.0
*■Tart, apple, w/apricot glaze	1	147	0.7	0	4.2
*■Yogurt, lemon-lime	1 serv.	84	1.2	3	12.8
Pie Crust Shells					
Mrs. Smith's 9"	⅛ shell	90	5.0	0	50.0
Pet-Ritz 9⅝"	⅙ shell	110	11.0	7	57.3
Pet-Ritz, Graham Cracker	⅙ shell	110	8.0	7	49.1

■ Contains less than 20% fat   57   * See page xxxii

Item	PORTION	CAL-ORIES	FAT GRAMS	CHOLES-TEROL	% OF FAT
Pie Crust Shell Mix, Flako	1 serving	245	15.0	9	55.1
Pie Fillings					
Comstock Fruit Pie Fillings (Lite)					
■ Apple	3.5 oz.	80	0.0	0	0.0
■ Blueberry	3.5 oz.	75	0.0	0	0.0
■ Cherry	3.5 oz.	75	0.0	0	0.0
■ Pumpkin Pie mix, Libby's	½ cup	105	0.0	0	0.0
Puddings					
Banana, canned, Town House	5 oz.	160	5.0	1	28.1
Bread					
Without raisins	1 cup	248	8.1	–	29.4
*■ Raisin Bread	1	74	0.5	2	6.0
Butterscotch, canned, Town House	5 oz.	160	5.0	1	28.1
Chocolate, prepared	½ cup	189	7.4	12	35.2
■Chocolate, instant, prepared w/milk from mix	½ cup	162	3.2	14	17.7
Chocolate Tapioca, prepared, Jell-O Americana	½ cup	169	4.7	16	25.0
Custard, baked	½ cup	95	3.2	90	30.3
*■Custard, cafe au lait	1	71	0.1	2	1.2
Egg custard, golden, prepared, Jell-O Americana	½ cup	162	5.3	80	29.4
Lemon					
■ Canned, Royal	½ cup	151	2.3	–	13.7
Instant, prepared, Jell-O	½ cup	76	2.0	–	23.7
Mousse, unflavored, prepared, Knorr	½ cup	80	5.0	5	56.2

Item	PORTION	CAL-ORIES	FAT GRAMS	CHOLES-TEROL	% OF FAT
Mousse, amaretto, prepared, Estee	½ cup	70	3.0	0	38.6
Mousse, cheesecake, Weight Watchers	½ cup	60	2.0	–	30.0
Mousse, chocolate					
Homemade	½ cup	217	12.5	144	51.8
Frozen, Weight Watchers	5 oz.	340	12.0	10	31.8
Mix, prepared					
Estee	½ cup	70	3.0	0	38.6
Knorr, dark or milk	½ cup	90	5.0	5	50.0
Lite Whip					
Made w/skim milk	½ cup	70	2.0	0	25.7
Made w/whole milk	½ cup	80	3.0	0	33.7
Weight Watchers, regular or white almond	½ cup	60	3.0	–	45.0
Mousse, vanilla, Lite Whip, made w/whole milk	½ cup	70	3.0	5	38.6
Pistachio, instant, prepared, from mix, Jell-O	½ cup	82	2.0	–	21.9
■Rice, with raisins	½ cup	193	4.0	15	18.6
Tapioca	½ cup	111	4.1	80	33.2
Vanilla, instant, prepared, from mix, Jell-O	½ cup	76	2.0	–	23.7
Other Desserts					
Baklava, homemade	1 oz.	112	8.2	20	65.9
Brownie (from mix)	1	130	5.0	–	35.0

■ Contains less than 20% fat   59

Item	PORTION	CAL-ORIES	FAT GRAMS	CHOLES-TEROL	% OF FAT
Cobbler					
Apple	1	211	9.8	0	41.9
Frozen, Pet-Ritz	4.3 oz.	290	9.0	–	27.9
Blackberry, frozen, Pet-Ritz	4.3 oz.	270	10.0	–	33.3
*■ Blueberry me-ringue	1	127	0.3	0	2.1
Peach, frozen, Pet-Ritz	4.3 oz.	260	10.0	–	25.0
Cream Puff, w/custard whipped cream	1	245	14.6	–	53.6
Dumpling, apple, fro-zen, Pepperidge Farm	1	281	17.0	–	54.4
Eclair					
Whipped cream filling & choco-late icing	1	296	25.0	–	76.0
Rich's, w/chocolate icing	1	240	14.0	–	52.5
W/custard filling & chocolate icing	1	251	13.1	152	47.0
*■Floating Island, w/strawberry sauce	1	110	0.4	0	3.2
■Jell-O, prepared	½ cup	61	0.0	0	0.0
Strudel, apple					
*■ Homemade	1	93	0.3	0	2.9
Frozen, Pepperidge Farm	1	240	11.0	–	41.2
*■Trifle, chocolate	1	69	1.5	1	19.3
Turnover					
Frozen, Pepperidge Farm					
Apple	1	300	17.0	–	51.0
Blueberry or cherry	1	310	19.0	–	55.2

Item	PORTION	CALORIES	FAT GRAMS	CHOLESTEROL	% OF FAT
Refrigerated, Pillsbury	2 oz.	170	8.0	5	42.4
Toppings					
■Butterscotch Smucker's	2 tb.	104	0.?	0	0.8
■ Regular	2 tb.	140	1.0	–	6.4
■ Special recipe	2 tb.	160	3.0	–	16.9
■Cherry	2 tb.	98	0.1	0	0.9
Chocolate fudge, Hershey	2 tb.	128	5.0	0	35.2
Cool Whip, non-dairy					
Regular	2 tb.	27	2.1	0	70.7
Xtra Creamy	2 tb.	31	2.4	–	69.7
*■Creme	1 tb.	21	0.0	0	0.0
Fudge, hot, Smucker's					
Regular or toffee	2 tb.	110	4.0	–	32.7
Special recipe	2 tb.	150	5.0	–	30.0
■Fudge, sweet, Orchard Farms	1 tsp.	16	0.0	0	0.0
Hot fudge	2 tb.	128	5.0	0	35.2
■Lemon sauce	2 tb.	42	0.3	1	6.4
■Marshmallow Creme, Kraft	1 oz.	89	0.0	0	0.0
■Pecans in syrup, Smucker's	2 tb.	130	1.0	–	6.9
■Pineapple	2 tb.	97	0.1	0	0.9
■Raisin sauce	2 tb.	71	1.0	0	12.7
■Strawberry	2 tb.	93	0.1	0	0.9
■Swiss milk chocolate	2 tb.	140	1.0	–	6.4
■Syrup, Chocolate, thin type	2 tb.	92	0.8	0	7.8
Syrup, Chocolate Fudge, Hershey	2 tb.	128	5.0	0	35.2
Whipped topping, non-dairy from can	2 tb.	23	1.9	0	74.3

■ Contains less than 20% fat

* See page xxxii

Item	PORTION	CAL-ORIES	FAT GRAMS	CHOLES-TEROL	% OF FAT
Whipped topping, non-dairy, frozen	2 tb.	30	2.4	0	72.0

EGGS, EGG DISHES & EGG SUBSTITUTES

Eggs
Chicken
■ White only, fresh, raw	1	16	0.0	0	0.0
Yolk only, fresh, raw	1	61	5.2	213	76.7
Fried, in butter	1	95	6.8	219	69.4
Hard cooked	1	80	5.3	213	61.1
Poached, in salt water	1	80	5.3	212	60.0
Scrambled w/milk, in butter	1	110	7.6	238	66.4
Soft cooked	1	80	5.3	213	61.1
Duck, whole, fresh, raw	1	111	8.3	530	67.2
Goose, whole, fresh, raw	1	266	19.1	–	64.6
Quail, whole, fresh, raw	1	14	1.0	76	64.2
Turkey, fresh	1	135	9.4	–	62.7

Egg Substitutes
■Egg Beaters, Fleischmann's	¼ cup	25	0.0	0	0.0
■Healthy Choice	¼ cup	30	0.0	0	0.0
■Morning Star, Better 'n Eggs	¼ cup	30	0.0	0	0.0
Second Nature	2 oz.	60	2.0	0	30.0
■The Right Egg	¼ cup	30	0.0	0	0.0
Tofutti Egg Watchers	¼ cup	50	2.0	0	36.0

■ Contains less than 20% fat

Item	PORTION	CAL-ORIES	FAT GRAMS	CHOLES-TEROL	% OF FAT
Egg Dishes					
Crepe, plain shell	1	80	2.7	71	30.3
* Frittata, no choles-terol	1	96	3.1	0	29.1
Omelet					
Homemade	3 eggs	287	21.6	639	67.7
Frozen, Great Starts, Swanson, w/cheese sauce & ham	1 (7 oz.)	390	29.0	–	66.9
Quiche	6 oz.	395	26.9	215	61.2
Scrambled, frozen, Downyflake, ham w/hash browns	1 (6.25 oz.)	360	26.0	–	65.0
Scrambled, frozen, Great Starts, Swanson					
& bacon, w/home fries	1 (5.6 oz.)	340	26.0	–	68.8
w/home fries	1 (4.6 oz.)	260	19.0	–	65.8
& sausage, w/hash browns	1 (6.5 oz.)	430	34.0	–	71.2

FAST FOODS

Item	PORTION	CAL-ORIES	FAT GRAMS	CHOLES-TEROL	% OF FAT
Arby's					
Apple turnover	1 serv.	310	21.0	0	61.0
Chicken breast					
Roasted	1 serv.	254	7.0	196	24.8
Sandwich	1 serv.	592	27.0	57	41.0
Chicken club sand-wich	1 serv.	621	32.0	108	46.4
Chicken salad crois-sant	1 serv.	460	36.0	111	70.4
French fries	1 serv.	211	8.0	6	34.1
Ham/cheese sand-wich, hot	1 serv.	353	13.0	50	33.1

Item	PORTION	CAL-ORIES	FAT GRAMS	CHOLES-TEROL	% OF FAT
Roast beef					
Junior	1 serv.	218	8.0	20	33.0
King	1 serv.	467	19.0	49	36.6
Super	1 serv.	501	22.0	40	39.5
Roast turkey deluxe	1 serv.	375	17.0	39	40.8
Shake					
Chocolate	10.6-oz. serv.	384	11.0	32	25.8
Vanilla	8.8-oz. serv.	295	10.0	30	30.5
Potato					
■ Baked, plain,	1 serv.	290	1.0	0	3.1
Super-stuffed, deluxe	1 serv.	648	38.0	72	52.8
Potato cakes	1 serv.	204	12.2	0	53.0
Arthur Treacher					
Chicken fillet, fried	1 serv.	369	22.0	65	53.6
Chicken sandwich	1 serv.	413	19.0	3	41.4
Chips (french fries)	1 serv.	276	13.0	1	42.4
Chowder	1 serv.	112	5.0	9	40.2
Coleslaw	1 serv.	123	8.0	7	58.5
Fish, fried	2 pieces	355	20.0	56	50.7
Fish sandwich	1 serv.	440	24.0	42	49.1
Krunch Pup	1 serv.	203	15.0	25	66.5
Shrimp, fried	1 serv.	381	24.0	93	56.7
Burger King					
■Bagel, plain	1 serv.	272	6.0	29	20.0
Bagel w/cream cheese	1 serv.	370	16.0	58	39.0
BK Broiler chicken Sandwich	1 serv.	379	18.0	53	42.7
Cheeseburger					
Single	1 serv.	317	15.0	48	42.6
Double	1 serv.	523	28.2	96	48.5
Chicken sandwich	1 serv.	685	40.0	82	52.4

■ Contains less than 20% fat   64

Item	PORTION	CAL-ORIES	FAT GRAMS	CHOLES-TEROL	% OF FAT
Chicken Tenders	6	204	10.0	47	44.1
Chocolate, hot	1 serv.	131	4.0	1	27.5
Croissanwich					
Regular	1 serv.	315	20.0	222	57.1
Egg/ham/cheese	1 serv.	335	20.0	241	53.7
Meat/egg/cheese	1 serv.	335	24.0	227	64.5
Sausage/egg/cheese	1 serv.	538	41.0	268	68.6
Danish	1 serv.	500	36.0	6	64.8
Dressing, Italian, re-duced calorie	1 serv.	170	18.0	0	95.3
Fish sandwich w/tartar sauce	1 serv.	495	25.0	57	45.5
French fries, regular serving	1 serv.	341	20.0	21	52.7
French toast					
w/bacon	1 serv.	469	30.0	73	57.6
w/sausage	1 serv.	635	46.0	115	65.2
Ham & cheese sand-wich	1 serv.	547	29.9	–	49.2
Hamburger, single	1 serv.	310	12.0	–	34.8
Onion rings, regular	1 serv.	274	16.0	0	52.5
Pie, apple	1 serv.	328	13.9	–	38.1
Salad					
Chef	1 serv.	178	9.0	103	45.5
Chicken, w/o Dressing	1 serv.	320	12.0	49	33.8
Garden Salad w/o Dressing	1 serv.	95	5.0	15	47.4
■ Side salad w/diet dressing	1 serv.	42	0.0	0	0
w/regular dress-ing	1 serv.	332	22.0	10	54.0
Scrambled Eggs					
Regular	1 serv.	468	30.0	370	57.7
w/bacon	1 serv.	536	36.0	378	60.4
w/sausage	1 serv.	702	52.0	420	66.6

■ Contains less than 20% fat

Item	PORTION	CAL-ORIES	FAT GRAMS	CHOLES-TEROL	% OF FAT
Shake					
Chocolate	1 serv.	326	10.0	31	27.6
Vanilla	1 serv.	321	10.0	31	28.0
Whaler Sandwich	1 serv.	488	27.0	84	50.0
Whopper					
Regular	1 serv.	669	38.0	–	51.1
w/cheese	1 serv.	761	45.1	–	53.3
Double	1 serv.	890	53.0	–	53.6
Double, w/cheese	1 serv.	975	65.3	–	60.3
Whopper Jr					
Regular	1 serv.	370	18.0	–	43.8
w/cheese	1 serv.	364	20.0	52	49.4
Carls JR					
Bacon & cheese potato, baked	1 (14.1 oz.)	650	34.0	45	47.1
Broccoli soup, cream of	1 (6 oz.)	140	6.0	22	38.6
Chicken sandwich					
■ Charbroiler BBQ	1 (6.3 oz.)	320	5.0	50	14.1
Charbroiler Club	1	510	22.0	85	38.8
Chocolate cake	1 serv.	380	20.0	70	47.4
Chocolate chip cookie	1 serv. (2.2 oz.)	330	13.0	0	35.5
Famous Star hamburger	1 serv.	530	32.0	70	54.3
Fish filet sandwich	1 serv.	570	27.0	40	42.6
Hash brown potato nuggets	1 serv.	170	9.0	10	47.6
Hot cakes, w/syrup & butter	1 serv.	480	15.0	15	28.1
■Lite potato, baked	1 serv.	250	3.0	0	10.8
Roast beef sandwich, w/swiss, California	1 serv.	360	8.0	130	20.0
Sour cream & chive potato, baked	1 serv.	350	13.0	10	33.4

Item	PORTION	CAL-ORIES	FAT GRAMS	CHOLES-TEROL	% OF FAT
Super Star hamburger	1 serv.	780	50.0	155	57.7
Western bacon cheeseburger, regular	1 serv.	630	33.0	105	47.1
Zucchini, fried	1 serv.	300	16.0	10	48.0
Church's					
Apple pie	1 serv.	300	19.0	–	57.0
Chicken, fried					
Breast	1 serv.	278	17.3	–	56.0
Leg	1 serv.	147	8.6	–	52.7
Thigh	1 serv.	306	21.6	–	63.5
Wing	1 serv.	303	19.7	–	58.5
Chicken nuggets, spicy	6 pieces	312	17.0	–	49.0
Corn, on cob, buttered	1 serv.	237	9.3	–	35.3
French fries, regular	1 serv. (3 oz.)	138	5.5	–	35.9
D' Lites					
Chicken fillet sandwich	1 serv.	280	11.0	45	35.4
■Chocolate d' lite	1 serv.	203	4.0	16	17.7
Fish fillet sandwich	1 serv.	390	21.0	95	48.5
Junior d' lite	1 serv.	200	7.0	55	31.5
Vegetarian sandwich	1 serv.	270	14.0	0	46.7
Dairy Queen					
Banana Split	1 serv.	535	14.9	57	25.1
Braizer					
Cheese dog	1 serv.	325	18.7	–	51.8
Chili dog	1 serv.	327	19.8	–	54.5
Hamburger, regular	1 serv.	257	8.9	–	31.2
Hot Dog	1 serv.	273	15.0	–	49.5
w/cheese	1 serv.	319	14.0	–	39.5

■ Contains less than 20% fat 67

Item	PORTION	CAL-ORIES	FAT GRAMS	CHOLES-TEROL	% OF FAT
Big Braizer					
Deluxe hamburger	1 serv.	470	24.0	–	45.9
Regular hamburger	1 serv.	454	22.9	–	45.4
w/cheese	1 serv.	554	30.0	–	48.7
Super Braizer					
Cheese dog	1 serv.	587	35.6	–	54.6
Chili dog	1 serv.	533	31.7	–	53.5
Hamburger	1 serv.	793	48.6	–	55.1
Hot dog	1 serv.	518	30.0	–	52.1
Brownie, hot fudge	1 serv.	577	22.2	–	34.6
Chicken sandwich	1 serv.	670	41.0	75	55.1
Fish sandwich					
Plain	1 serv.	401	17.0	–	38.1
w/cheese	1 serv.	440	21.0	60	43.0
Freeze					
Regular	1 serv.	516	12.9	–	22.5
Mr. Misty	1 serv.	493	11.8	–	21.5
French fries					
Small	1 serv.	197	9.9	–	45.2
Large	1 serv.	315	15.8	–	45.1
Hamburger w/cheese, triple	1 serv.	820	50.0	145	54.9
Ice cream bar, Buster	1 serv.	389	21.9	–	50.7
Ice cream cone bar, Dilly	1 serv.	241	15.0	–	56.0
Ice cream cone					
Small	1 serv.	109	3.0	–	24.8
Medium	1 serv.	227	6.9	–	27.4
Ice cream float	1 serv.	328	7.9	–	21.7
Ice cream sandwich	1 serv.	140	4.9	24	31.5
Ice cream sundae, chocolate					
Small	1 serv.	168	3.9	–	20.9
Medium	1 serv.	309	5.1	–	24.8
Malt, Chocolate	med.	600	20.0	–	30.0
Onion rings	1 serv.	301	17.0	–	50.8

■ Contains less than 20% fat   68

Item	PORTION	CAL-ORIES	FAT GRAMS	CHOLES-TEROL	% OF FAT
Denny's (See Coffee Shop, p. 186)					
Bacon, lettuce & to-mato sandwich	1 serv.	542	33.0	41	54.8
Chef salad	1 serv.	263	22.0	364	73.3
Chicken breast sand-wich	1 serv.	830	47.0	124	51.0
Chicken steak, fried	1 serv.	606	62.0	87	92.1
Chicken stir fry	1 serv.	435	43.0	104	89.0
Chicken strips	4 oz.	240	10.0	–	37.0
Cinnamon roll	1	450	14.0	–	27.0
Club sandwich	1 serv.	590	20.0	65	51.3
Denny burger	1 serv.	537	44.0	319	73.4
Denny's chef salad	1 serv.	263	22.0	364	73.3
Denny's taco salad (w/fried taco shell)	1 serv.	953	50.0	–	47.0
Eggs Benedict	1 serv.	658	36.0	–	27.0
French toast w/butter and powdered sugar	2 slices	729	56.0	–	69.0
Grand Slam	1 serv.	1005	59.0	698	52.3
Patty melt	1 serv.	657	45.0	186	61.6
Waffles	1	261	10.0	–	34.0
Turkey sandwich, sliced	1 serv.	445	26.0	53	52.6
Waffles	1	261	10.0	?	34.0
Domino's Pizza					
Cheese (16″ pie)	2 slices	376	10.0	18	23.9
Deluxe (16″ pie)	2 slices	498	20.4	40	36.9
Double cheese/pepperoni (16″ pie)	2 slices	545	25.3	48	41.8
Ham (16″ pie)	2 slices	417	11.0	26	23.7
Pepperoni (16″ pie)	2 slices	460	17.5	28	34.2
Sausage & mushroom (16″ pie)	2 slices	430	15.7	28	32.9

■ Contains less than 20% fat

Item	PORTION	CAL-ORIES	FAT GRAMS	CHOLES-TEROL	% OF FAT
Veggie (16″ pie)	2 slices	498	18.5	36	33.4
Godfather's					
Cheese					
■ Mini, original	2 slices	380	8.0	16	18.9
Large, original					
Regular	2 slices	594	18.0	40	30.6
Hot slice	2 slices	740	22.0	50	26.8
Stuffed, large	2 slices	762	32.0	64	37.8
Thin crust, large	2 slices	456	14.0	32	27.6
Combo					
Large, regular	2 slices	874	38.0	72	39.1
Stuffed, large	2 slices	1042	52.0	96	44.9
Thin crust, large	2 slices	672	32.0	54	42.9
Hardees					
Apple turnover	1 serv.	270	12.0	0	40.0
Big Cookie	1 serv.	250	13.0	5	46.8
Big Country Breakfast					
w/ham	1 serv.	620	33.0	325	47.9
w/sausage	1 serv.	850	57.0	340	60.3
Biscuit					
Bacon	1 serv.	360	21.0	10	52.5
Bacon, egg & cheese	1 serv.	460	28.0	165	54.9
Chicken	1 serv.	430	22.0	45	46.0
Country ham & egg	1 serv.	400	22.0	175	49.5
& gravy	1 serv.	440	26.0	15	53.2
Ham w/egg	1 serv.	370	19.0	160	46.2
Rise & Shine, w/Canadian bacon	1 serv.	320	18.0	0	50.6
Sausage w/egg	1 serv.	490	31.0	170	56.9
Cheeseburger					
Plain	1 serv.	320	14.0	30	39.4
Quarter-pound	1 serv.	500	29.0	70	52.2

Item	PORTION	CAL-ORIES	FAT GRAMS	CHOLES-TEROL	% OF FAT
Chicken fillet sand-wich	1 serv.	370	13.0	55	31.6
Chicken, grilled, sandwich	1 serv.	310	9.0	60	26.1
Chicken Stix, 6-piece	1 serv.	210	9.0	35	38.6
Fisherman's Fillet, sandwich	1 serv.	500	24.0	70	43.2
Hamburger					
Plain	1 serv.	270	10.0	20	33.3
Big Deluxe	1 serv.	500	30.0	70	54.0
Hot ham & cheese sandwich	1 serv.	330	12.0	65	32.7
Pancakes, 3					
■ Plain	1 serv.	280	1.0	2	3.2
w/sausage patty	1 serv.	430	16.0	40	33.5
Potato					
French fries, regu-lar	1 serv.	230	11.0	0	43.0
Hash Rounds	1 serv.	230	14.0	0	54.8
Roast beef sandwich, big	1 serv.	300	11.0	45	33.0
Salads					
Chef	1 serv.	240	15.0	115	56.2
■ Chicken & pasta	1 serv.	230	3.0	55	11.7
Shake					
■ Chocolate	1 serv.	460	8.0	45	15.6
■ Strawberry	1 serv.	440	8.0	40	16.4
Vanilla	1 serv.	400	9.0	50	20.2
■Syrup	1 serv.	120	0.0	0	0.0
Turkey club sandwich	1 serv.	390	15.0	70	34.6
Jack-in-the-Box					
Apple turnover	1 serv.	411	23.9	17	52.3
Breakfast Jack	1 serv.	301	13.1	182	39.2
Cheese nachos	1 serv.	571	36	37	56.7
Cheeseburger	1 serv.	323	15.0	42	41.8
Chicken fajita	1 serv.	292	8.0	34	24.7

■ Contains less than 20% fat   71

Item	PORTION	CAL-ORIES	FAT GRAMS	CHOLES-TEROL	% OF FAT
French fries	1 serv.	271	15.0	14	49.8
Hamburger					
Regular	1 serv.	262	10.5	25	36.1
Jumbo Jack	1 serv.	551	28.5	81	46.5
Moby Jack sandwich	1 serv.	452	26	56	51.8
Mushroom burger	1 serv.	470	24.0	64	45.9
Onion rings	1 serv.	351	22.7	24	58.2
Pancake breakfast	1 serv.	624	27.3	88	39.4
Pita, club	1 serv.	277	8.0	43	25.9
Sausage crescent	1 serv.	584	43.0	187	66.3
Scrambled egg break-fast	1 serv.	718	43.5	259	54.5
Shake					
■ Chocolate	1 serv.	325	4.4	26	12.2
■ Vanilla	1 serv.	320	4.4	25	12.4
Taco					
Regular	1 serv.	187	10.7	21	51.5
Super	1 serv.	285	17.2	37	54.3
Taco salad	1 serv.	377	24.0	–	57.3
KFC					
■Barbecue sauce	1 oz.	35	.6	0	15.4
Biscuit, buttermilk	1	235	11.7	1	44.8
Breast, center					
Original	1	283	15.3	92	48.7
Extra Tasty Crispy	1	344	21.0	80	54.9
Lite 'N Crispy	1	220	11.9	57	48.7
Chicken Littles sand-wich	1 serv.	169	10.1	18	53.8
Chicken nugget	1	46	2.9	12	56.7
Coleslaw	1 serv.	119	6.6	5	49.9
Colonel's Chicken Sandwich	1 serv.	482	27.3	47	50.9
■Corn-on-the-cob	1 serv.	176	3.1	0	16.1
Drumstick					
Extra Tasty Crispy	1	205	14.0	72	61.5
Lite 'N Crispy	1	121	7.0	51	52.1

■ Contains less than 20% fat

Item	PORTION	CAL-ORIES	FAT GRAMS	CHOLES-TEROL	% OF FAT
French fries, regular	1 serv.	244	11.9	2	43.9
Gravy, chicken	1 serv.	59	3.7	2	56.4
Honey sauce	.5 oz.	49	0.0	0	0.0
Hot wings	1	63	4.0	25	57.1
■Potatoes, mashed	1 serv.	59	0.6	0	9.1
Side breast					
Extra Tasty Crispy	1	379	27.0	77	64.1
Lite 'N Crispy	1	204	12.4	53	54.7
■Sweet & sour sauce	1 oz.	58	0.6	0	9.3
Thigh					
Original	1	294	19.7	123	60.3
Extra Tasty Crispy	1	414	31.0	112	67.4
Lite 'N Crispy	1	246	16.7	80	61.1
Wing					
Original	1	178	11.7	64	59.1
Extra Tasty Crispy	1	254	18.6	67	65.9
Long John Silver					
Catfish filet	1 (2.5 oz.)	180	11.0	25	55.0
Chicken flank	1 piece	110	6.0	15	49.1
Children's meal	1 serv.	510	24.0	30	42.3
Dinner	3 pieces	830	39.0	55	42.3
Clam					
Breaded	1 serv.	240	12.0	2	45.0
Dinner	1 serv.	980	45.0	15	41.3
Clam chowder, w/cod	7 oz.	140	6.0	20	38.6
■Cod					
Baked	1 serv.	150	0.0	135	0.0
Delight	1 serv.	180	1.0	135	5.0
Supreme	1 serv.	190	4.0	135	18.9
Broiled	1 serv.	160	2.0	110	11.2
Coleslaw, drained	1 serv.	140	6.0	15	38.6
■Corn-on-the-cob	1 serv.	85	1.0	0	10.0
Fish, battered	1 piece	150	8.0	30	48.0
Fish & chicken entree	1 serv.	870	40.0	70	41.4
Fish & chicken plank, children's meal	1 serv.	550	26.0	45	42.5

■ Contains less than 20% fat

Item	PORTION	CAL-ORIES	FAT GRAMS	CHOLES-TEROL	% OF FAT
Fish dinner	3 pieces	960	44.0	100	41.2
Homestyle	3 pieces	880	42.0	75	42.9
Fish & fries entree	2 pieces	660	30.0	60	40.9
Fish sandwich, home-style	1 serv.	510	22.0	45	38.8
Fish sandwich platter, homestyle	1 serv.	870	38.0	55	39.3
Flounder, broiled	1 piece	180	8.0	70	40.0
Gumbo, w/cod & shrimp bobs	7 oz.	120	8.0	25	60.0
Hushpuppie	1 piece	70	2.0	0	25.7
Pecan pie	1 serv.	530	25.0	70	42.4
Potato					
■ Baked, plain	1 serv.	150	0.0	0	0.0
Fries	1 serv.	220	10.0	4	40.9
■Rice pilaf	1 serv.	150	2.0	0	12.0
Salad					
Ocean chef	1 serv.	250	9.0	80	32.4
■ Side	1 serv.	20	0.0	0	0.0
Salmon, broiled	1 piece	180	4.0	70	20.0
Seafood platter entree	1 serv.	970	46.0	70	42.7
Shrimp, battered	1 piece	40	3.0	10	67.5
Dinner	6 pieces	740	37.0	90	45.0
Shrimp, breaded	1 serv.	190	10.0	40	47.4
Feast	13 pieces	880	41.0	90	41.9
Shrimp & fish dinner	1 serv.	770	37.0	80	43.2
Shrimp scampi, baked	1 serv.	160	37.0	80	43.2
■Sweet & sour sauce	1 pkt.	60	0.0	0	0.0
Tartar sauce	1 pkt.	80	3.0	–	33.7
Vegetables, mixed	1 serv.	60	2.0	0	30.0
McDonald's					
Big Mac	1 serv.	560	32.4	103	52.1
Biscuit					
w/bacon, egg & cheese	1 serv.	440	26.4	253	54.0
w/biscuit spread	1 serv.	260	12.7	1	43.9

■ Contains less than 20% fat   74

Item	PORTION	CAL-ORIES	FAT GRAMS	CHOLES-TEROL	% OF FAT
w/sausage & egg	1 serv.	520	34.5	275	59.7
Cheeseburger	1 serv.	310	13.8	53	40.1
Chicken McNuggets	1 serv. (4 oz.)	290	16.3	65	50.6
Cookies					
Chocolate chip	1 serv.	330	15.6	4	42.5
McDonaldland	1 serv.	290	9.2	0	28.5
Danish					
Apple	1	390	17.9	25	41.3
Cheese, iced	1	390	21.8	47	50.3
Cinnamon raisin	1	440	21.0	34	42.9
Dressings					
French	½ oz.	58	5.2	0	80.7
Reduced calorie	½ oz.	40	1.9	0	42.7
Ranch	½ oz.	83	8.6	5	93.2
Vinaigrette, lite	½ oz.	15	0.5	0	30.0
Egg McMuffin	1 serv.	290	11.2	226	34.8
Eggs, scrambled	1 serv.	140	9.8	399	63.0
Filet-O-Fish sandwich	1 serv.	440	26.1	50	53.4
Hamburger	1 serv.	260	9.5	37	32.9
Hot cakes w/butter & syrup	1 serv.	410	9.2	21	20.2
McChicken sandwich	1 serv.	490	28.6	43	52.5
McD.L.T.	1 serv.	580	36.8	109	57.1
McLean DeLuxe	1 serv.	320	10.0	60	28.1
Milk Shake					
Chocolate	1 serv.	390	10.6	41	24.5
Vanilla	1 serv.	350	10.2	41	26.2
■ Low fat					
Chocolate or Strawberry	1 serv.	320	2.2	–	6.2
Vanilla	1 serv.	290	2.2	–	6.8
Muffin, English, w/butter	1	170	4.6	9	24.3
Pie, apple	1 serv.	260	14.8	6	51.2

■ Contains less than 20% fat　　75

Item	PORTION	CAL-ORIES	FAT GRAMS	CHOLES-TEROL	% OF FAT
Potatoes					
French fries, small	1 serv.	220	11.5	9	47.0
Hashbrown	1 serv.	130	7.3	9	50.5
Quarter Pounder	1 serv.	410	20.7	86	45.4
w/cheese	1 serv.	520	29.2	118	50.3
Salads					
Chef	1 serv.	230	13.6	128	53.2
Chicken, chunky	1 serv.	140	3.4	78	21.8
Garden	1 serv.	110	6.8	83	55.6
Side	1 serv.	60	3.3	41	49.5
Sauces					
■ Barbecue	1.1 oz.	50	0.5	0	9.0
■ Honey	½ oz.	45	0.0	0	0.0
Hot mustard	1 oz.	70	2.0	2	25.7
■ Sweet & sour	1.1 oz.	60	0.2	0	3.0
Sausage	1 serv.	180	16.3	48	81.5
Sausage McMuffin	1 serv.	370	21.9	64	53.3
w/egg	1 serv.	440	27.4	263	56.0
■Sorbet, orange	3 oz.	106	0.0	–	0.0
Sundae					
Hot caramel	1 serv.	340	9.1	35	24.1
Hot fudge	1 serv.	310	9.4	28	27.3
Strawberry	1 serv.	280	7.3	27	23.5
■Yogurt, frozen					
Cone	1 serv.	100	0.7	3	6.3
Low-fat	3 oz.	100	1.0	–	9.0
Roy Rogers					
Biscuit	1	231	12.1	0	47.1
Breakfast crescent sandwich					
Regular	1 serv.	408	27.3	207	60.2
w/bacon	1 serv.	446	29.7	212	59.9
w/sausage	1 serv.	564	42.0	248	67.0
Cheeseburger	1 serv.	525	29.0	76	49.7
w/bacon	1 serv.	552	33.0	83	53.8
Chicken					
Breast	1	412	23.7	118	51.8

■ Contains less than 20% fat

Item	PORTION	CAL-ORIES	FAT GRAMS	CHOLES-TEROL	% OF FAT
Breast & wing	1	604	36.5	165	54.4
Leg	1	140	8.0	40	51.4
Thigh	1	296	19.5	85	59.3
Thigh & leg	1	436	27.5	125	56.8
Wing	1	192	12.8	47	60.0
Chicken nuggets	1 piece	48	3.0	10	56.2
Egg & biscuit platter					
Regular	1 serv.	557	34.0	417	54.9
w/bacon	1 serv.	607	39.0	424	57.8
w/ham	1 serv.	605	36.0	437	53.5
w/sausage	1 serv.	713	49.0	458	61.8
Hamburger	1 serv.	472	25.0	64	47.7
Bar Burger	1 serv.	573	31.0	96	48.7
Pancake platter, w/syrup & butter	1 serv.	386	13.0	51	30.3
w/bacon	1 serv.	436	17.0	58	35.1
w/ham	1 serv.	434	15.0	71	31.1
w/sausage	1 serv.	542	28.0	92	46.5
Potato, french fries, regular	1 serv.	320	16.0	13	45.0
Roast beef sandwich					
Plain					
Regular	1 serv.	350	11.0	58	28.3
Large	1 serv.	373	11.9	82	28.7
w/cheese					
Regular	1 serv.	403	15.0	70	33.5
Large	1 serv.	427	17.0	94	35.8
Salad bar					
Bacon bits	1 tb.	33	1.0	–	27.3
■ Beets, sliced	¼ cup	18	0.0	–	0.0
■ Carrots, shredded	¼ cup	12	0.0	–	0.0
Cheese, cheddar	¼ cup	112	9.0	–	72.3
■ Croutons	1 tb.	35	0.0	–	0.0
■ Cucumber	1 slice	0	0.0	–	0.0
Egg, chopped	1 tb.	27	2.0	–	66.7
■ Mushrooms	¼ cup	5	0.0	–	0.0

■ Contains less than 20% fat

Item	PORTION	CAL-ORIES	FAT GRAMS	CHOLES-TEROL	% OF FAT
■ Pea, green	¼ cup	7	0.0	–	0.0
Sunflower seeds	1 tb.	78	6.6	–	76.1
Salad dressing					
Bacon & tomato	1 tb.	68	6.0	–	79.4
Bleu cheese	1 tb.	75	8.0	–	96.0
1000 Island	1 tb.	80	8.0	–	90.0
Lite, Italian	1 tb.	35	3.0	–	77.1
Sundae					
Caramel	1 serv.	293	8.5	23	26.1
Hot fudge	1 serv.	337	12.5	186	33.4
Strawberry	1 serv.	216	7.1	23	29.6
Shakey's					
Chicken, fried, & potatoes	3 pieces	947	56.0	–	53.2
Ham & cheese, hot	1 serv.	550	21.0	–	34.4
Pizza					
Cheese, 12″ pie					
Homestyle pan crust	⅒ of pie	303	13.7	–	40.7
Thin crust	⅒ of pie	133	5.2	–	35.2
Pepperoni, 12″ pie					
Thick crust	⅒ of pie	185	6.4	–	31.1
Thin crust	⅒ of pie	148	6.9	–	41.9
Special, 12″ pie, homestyle	⅒ of pie	384	20.7	–	48.5
Potatoes, 15-pieces	1 serv.	950	36.0	–	34.1
Spaghetti w/meat sauce & garlic bread	1 serv.	940	33.0	–	31.6
Super hot hero	1 serv.	810	44.0	–	48.9
Taco Bell					
Burrito					
Bean, green sauce	1 serv.	351	10.1	9	25.9
Beef, red sauce	1 serv.	403	17.3	57	38.6

■ Contains less than 20% fat   78

Item	PORTION	CAL-ORIES	FAT GRAMS	CHOLES-TEROL	% OF FAT
Supreme, green sauce	1 serv.	407	17.5	33	38.7
Double beef	1 serv.	451	21.8	57	43.5
Cinnamon Crispas	1 serv.	259	15.3	0	53.2
Enchirito, red sauce	1 serv.	382	19.7	54	46.4
Fajita					
Chicken	1 serv.	225	10.2	44	40.8
Steak	1 serv.	234	10.9	14	41.9
Guacamole	¾ oz.	34	2.3	0	60.9
Meximelt	1 serv.	266	15.4	38	52.1
Nachos	1 serv.	346	18.5	9	48.1
Bellgrande	1 serv.	648	35.3	36	49.0
Pico De Gallo	1 oz.	8	0.2	0	22.5
Pintos & cheese	1 serv.	184	8.7	16	42.5
Pizza, Mexican	1 serv.	575	36.8	52	57.6
Ranch dressing	1 serv.	236	24.8	35	94.6
■Salsa	1 serv. (.3 oz.)	18	0.1	0	5.0
Sour cream	¾ oz.	46	4.4	–	86.1
Taco					
Regular	1 serv.	183	10.8	32	53.1
Bellgrande	1 serv.	355	23.1	56	58.6
Light	1 serv.	410	28.8	56	63.2
Soft, Supreme	1 serv.	275	16.3	32	53.3
Taco salad					
w/o shell w/salsa	1 serv.	502	31.3	80	56.1
Regular	1 serv.	941	61.3	80	58.6
w/o shell	1 serv.	520	31.4	80	54.3
Taco sauce	1 pkt.	2	0.1	0	45.0
Tostada, green sauce	1 serv.	237	11.1	16	42.1
Taco John's					
Burrito					
Bean	1 serv.	197	6.0	–	27.4
Beef	1 serv.	303	18.0	–	53.5
Chicken	1 serv.	227	10.0	–	39.6

■ Contains less than 20% fat

Item	PORTION	CAL-ORIES	FAT GRAMS	CHOLES-TEROL	% OF FAT
w/green chili	1 serv.	344	12.0	–	31.4
Combo	1 serv.	250	12.0	–	43.2
Smothered					
w/green chili	1 serv.	367	18.0	–	44.1
w/Texas chili	1 serv.	455	23.0	–	45.5
Super	1 serv.	389	16.0	–	37.0
w/chicken	1 serv.	366	14.0	–	34.4
Chimichanga	1 serv.	464	20.0	–	38.8
w/chicken	1 serv.	441	19.0	–	38.8
Mexican rice	8 oz.	340	8.0	–	21.2
Nachos	1 serv.	468	25.0	–	48.1
Super	1 serv.	669	39.0	–	52.5
Potato Ole, large	1 serv.	414	24.0	–	52.3
Taco	1 serv.	178	13.0	–	65.7
w/chicken	1 serv.	140	9.0	–	57.8
Soft shell	1 serv.	224	13.0	–	52.2
w/chicken	1 serv.	180	8.0	–	40.0
Taco Bravo	1 serv.	319	14.0	–	39.5
Super	1 serv.	361	19.0	–	47.4
Taco burger	1 serv.	281	14.0	–	44.8
Taco salad					
Regular					
w/o dressing	1 serv.	228	13.0	–	51.3
w/2-oz. dressing	1 serv.	359	24.0	–	60.2
Chicken					
w/o dressing	1 serv.	377	15.0	–	35.8
w/dressing	1 serv.	507	27.0	–	47.9
Wendy's					
Big Classic Double	1 serv.	680	39.0	155	51.6
Biscuit, buttermilk	1 serv.	320	17.0	0	47.8
Breakfast Sandwich	1 serv.	369	19.0	200	46.3
Cheeseburger					
Single	1 serv.	576	34.3	89	53.6
Double	1 serv.	796	48.1	156	54.4
Triple	1 serv.	1036	67.2	22	58.4
Chicken fried steak	1 serv.	580	41.0	95	63.6

■ Contains less than 20% fat   80

Item	PORTION	CALORIES	FAT GRAMS	CHOLESTEROL	% OF FAT
Chicken nuggets	1 serv.	290	21.0	55	65.2
Chicken sandwich on multigrain bun	1 serv.	320	10.0	59	28.1
Chili	1 serv.	228	7.5	25	29.6
Cottage cheese	½ cup	110	5.0	15	40.9
Danish	1 serv.	400	17.7	–	39.8
French fries	1 serv.	328	15.7	6	43.1
Frosty	1 serv.	393	16.0	45	36.6
Hamburger, single	1 serv.	472	26.0	68	49.6
Hamburger, double	1 serv.	667	39.2	125	52.9
Hamburger, triple	1 serv.	830	50.0	200	54.2
Omelet, ham/cheese/ mushroom	1 serv.	288	20.9	357	65.3
Potato					
■ Baked, plain	1 serv.	250	2.0	0	7.2
Baked with bacon/ cheese	1 serv.	579	30.1	22	46.8
Breakfast	1 serv.	360	22.0	20	55.0
Sausage patty	1 serv.	200	18.0	45	81.0
Scrambled eggs	2	190	12.0	450	56.8

FATS & OILS

Item	PORTION	CALORIES	FAT GRAMS	CHOLESTEROL	% OF FAT
Bacon rind	½ oz.	79	8.2	9	93.4
Beef fat	1 tb.	116	12.8	14	100.0
Butter					
Stick	1 tb.	102	11.5	31	100.0
Whipped	1 tb.	68	7.7	21	100.0
Butter, imitation					
■ Butter Buds, dry powder	½ tsp.	4	0.0	1	0.0
■ Butter Buds, pre- pared	1 tb.	6	0.0	0	0.0
■ Molly McButter	½ tsp.	4	0.0	0	0.0
Chicken fat	1 tb.	115	12.8	11	100.0

■ Contains less than 20% fat   81

Item	PORTION	CAL-ORIES	FAT GRAMS	CHOLES-TEROL	% OF FAT
Fat, Imitation					
Rokeach Neutral Nyafat	1 tb.	99	11.0	0	100.0
Margarine					
Regular	1 tb.	101	11.4	0	100.0
Fleischmann's	1 tb.	100	11.2	–	100.0
Mrs Filbert's, 100% Veg	1 tb.	100	11	0	99.0
Mazola	1 tb.	101	11.2	0	99.8
Nucoa	1 tb.	99	11.2	0	100.0
Nucoa Heart Beat	1 tb.	25	3.0	0	36.0
Parkay Spread, 70% Veg	1 tb.	88	9.7	0	99.2
Parkay	½ oz.	104	11.4	0	98.6
Promise Stick	1 tb.	90	10.0	0	100.0
Promise, soft	1 tb.	100	11.2	0	100.0
Margarine, light or diet, stick	1 tb.	50	5.6	0	100.0
Fleischmann's, Extra light	1 tb.	50	6.0	0	100.0
Fleischmann's, Light	1 tb.	81	8.1	0	90.0
Promise Extra Light spread	1 tb.	50	6.0	0	100.0
Weight Watchers, sweet, reduced cal., tub	1 tb.	50	6.0	0	100.0
Weight Watchers, salted, tub	1 tb.	60	7.3	0	100.0
Margarine, light or diet, tub					
Le Slim Cow	1 tb.	56	6.0	–	96.4
Nucoa Heart Smart	1 tb.	25	3.0	0	100.0
Promise, extra light,	1 tb.	50	6.0	0	100.0
Margarine, butter blend, regular					
Country Morning	1 tb.	90	10.0	0	100.0

■ Contains less than 20% fat

Item	PORTION	CAL-ORIES	FAT GRAMS	CHOLES-TEROL	% OF FAT
I Can't Believe It's Not Butter	1 tb.	90	10.0	0	100.0
Touch of Butter, stick	1 tb.	90	10.0	0	100.0
Touch of Butter, tub	1 tb.	50	6.0	0	100.0
Margarine, butter blend, light					
Country Morning	1 tb.	70	7.0	–	90.0
Margarine, diet, imitation, Mazola	1 tb.	48	5.4	0	100.0
Margarine, Liquid, Parkay	1 tb.	102	11.3	0	99.7
Oil, all types	1 tb.	121	13.6	0	100.0
Pam, non-stick spray	1 spray	2	0.2	0	90.0
Salt pork	½ oz.	106	11.4	12	96.8
Shortening, lard					
Regular	1 tb.	121	13.6	12	100.0
Shortening, Vegetable, Crisco	1 tb.	106	12.0	0	100.0

FISH & SHELLFISH

Item	PORTION	CAL-ORIES	FAT GRAMS	CHOLES-TEROL	% OF FAT
■Abalone, raw	3 oz.	89	0.6	72	6.0
Anchovy, canned, in oil, drained	3 fillets	21	1.2	12	90.0
Anchovy paste	1 tsp.	14	0.8	–	51.5
Bass					
Black Sea, raw	3 oz.	97	3.1	58	28.7
Striped, raw	3 oz.	82	2.0	68	21.9
White, raw	3 oz.	97	3.1	58	28.7
Bluefish, raw	3.5 oz.	105	3.6	50	30.8
Buffalofish	3 oz.	113	4.2	–	33.4
Butterfish, raw	3 oz.	124	6.8	55	49.3
■Calamari, raw (squid)	3 oz.	110	1.2	26	9.8
Calamari, fried	3 oz.	149	6.4	221	38.6
Carp, raw	3 oz.	108	4.8	56	40.0

Item	PORTION	CAL-ORIES	FAT GRAMS	CHOLES-TEROL	% OF FAT
Catfish, freshwater, raw	3 oz.	99	3.6	49	32.7
■Caviar, black and red	1 tb.	40	2.0	165	11.0
■Clams					
Canned, solids/liquids	3 oz.	44	0.5	27	10.2
Raw	3 oz.	63	0.8	29	11.4
■Cod, Atlantic					
Cooked	3 oz.	89	0.7	47	7.0
Dried	3 oz.	247	2.0	129	7.2
■Crab					
Blue, canned, drained	3 oz.	84	1.0	76	10.7
Blue, cooked	3 oz.	87	1.5	85	15.5
Dungeness, raw	3 oz.	73	0.8	50	9.8
King, cooked	3 oz.	82	1.3	45	14.2
Imitation, from Surimi	3 oz.	87	1.1	17	11.3
■Crayfish, raw	3 oz.	76	0.9	118	10.6
Croaker, white, raw	3 oz.	88	2.7	52	27.6
■Dolphinfish, raw	3 oz.	72	0.6	62	7.5
Eel, cooked	3 oz.	201	12.7	137	56.8
Fish sticks, frozen, cooked	1	76	3.4	31	40.2
Fish cake, frozen, cooked	3 oz.	231	10.4	95	40.5
■Flounder, cooked	3 oz.	100	1.3	58	11.7
■Gefilte fish	1 piece	70	1.0	–	13.0
■Grouper, raw	3 oz.	78	0.9	31	10.3
■Haddock					
Cooked	3 oz.	95	0.8	63	7.5
Smoked	3 oz.	99	0.8	65	7.2
■Halibut, cooked	3 oz.	119	2.5	35	18.9
Herring					
Raw	3 oz.	134	7.7	51	51.7
Pickled	3 oz.	223	15.3	51	61.7
■Lingcod, raw	3 oz.	72	0.9	44	·11.2

■ Contains less than 20% fat

Item	PORTION	CAL-ORIES	FAT GRAMS	CHOLES-TEROL	% OF FAT
Lobster					
Newburg	3 oz.	174	13.9	133	71.8
■ Northern, cooked	3 oz.	83	0.5	81	5.4
■ Spiny, raw	3 oz.	95	1.3	60	12.3
Mackerel					
Atlantic, cooked	3 oz.	223	15.1	64	60.9
Jack, canned, drained	3 oz.	133	5.4	67	36.5
Pacific, raw	3 oz.	100	3.2	42	28.8
■Mahi Mahi, fillet, raw	3 oz.	73	1.0	62	12.3
■Monkfish, raw	3 oz.	65	1.3	21	18.0
Mullet, striped, raw	3 oz.	100	3.2	42	28.8
Mussels					
Blue, raw	3 oz.	73	1.9	24	23.4
Canned	3.5 oz.	114	3.3	30	26.0
Orange Roughy, raw	3 oz.	107	6.0	17	50.4
Oysters, Eastern					
Canned	3 oz.	59	2.1	47	32.0
Fried	3 oz.	168	10.7	69	57.3
Raw	3 oz.	59	2.1	47	32.0
Oysters, Pacific, raw	3 oz.	69	2.0	–	26.0
■Perch, lake					
Raw	3 oz.	77	0.8	77	9.3
Cooked	3 oz.	100	1.0	98	9.0
■Perch, ocean					
Raw	3 oz.	80	1.4	36	15.7
Cooked	3 oz.	103	1.8	46	15.7
■Pickerel, raw	3 oz.	79	1.0	73	11.3
■Pike					
Blue, raw	3 oz.	79	1.0	73	11.3
Northern, raw	3 oz.	75	0.6	33	7.2
Walleye, raw	3 oz.	79	1.0	73	11.3
■Pollack, Atlantic, raw	3 oz.	78	0.8	60	9.2
Pompano, raw	3 oz.	139	8.1	43	52.4
■Rockfish, cooked	3 oz.	103	1.7	37	14.8
Salmon					
Atlantic, raw	3 oz.	121	5.4	47	40.1

■ Contains less than 20% fat

Item	PORTION	CAL-ORIES	FAT GRAMS	CHOLES-TEROL	% OF FAT
Coho, cooked	3 oz.	157	6.4	42	36.6
Pink, canned	3 oz.	118	5.1	–	38.8
Smoked (Lox)	3 oz.	100	3.7	20	33.3
Sockeye, canned	3 oz.	130	6.2	37	45.4
Sardine					
Atlantic, canned in oil	3½ oz.	200	11.0	17	50.4
Pacific, canned in tomato	3½ oz.	200	12.0	23	54.0
Scallops					
Sea or bay, cooked	3½ oz.	81	1.2	30	13.3
*■ Ceviche	3½ oz.	110	1.0	37	8.0
Fried, sea	3½ oz.	200	8.0	37	36.0
*■ Stir-fried	1 serv.	182	3.3	37	16.3
■ Imitation, from Surimi	3 oz.	84	0.3	19	3.2
■Sea Bass					
Raw	3 oz.	82	1.7	35	18.6
Cooked	3 oz.	105	2.2	45	18.8
Shark, raw	3 oz.	111	3.8	43	30.8
Shrimp					
Fried, breaded	3 oz.	206	10.4	151	45.4
■ Steamed, large	3 oz.	84	0.9	151	9.6
Smelt, rainbow, raw	3 oz.	82	2.1	60	23.0
■Snapper, raw	3 oz.	85	1.1	31	11.6
■Sole, fillet					
Raw	3 oz.	77	1.0	41	11.6
Cooked	3 oz.	100	1.3	58	11.7
Squid, fried	3 oz.	149	6.4	221	38.6
Sturgeon, cooked	3 oz.	115	4.4	–	34.4
Sucker, carp, cooked	3 oz.	138	6.1	71	39.7
■Surimi	3½ oz.	98	0.9	30	8.5
Sushi (fish, rice & seaweed)	3 oz.	106	3.5	23	29.7
Swordfish, raw	3 oz.	103	3.4	33	29.7
Trout					
Lake, raw	3 oz.	126	5.6	49	40.0

■ Contains less than 20% fat   86   * See page xxxii

Item	PORTION	CAL-ORIES	FAT GRAMS	CHOLES-TEROL	% OF FAT
Ocean, raw	3 oz.	126	5.6	49	40.0
Rainbow, raw	3 oz.	100	2.9	48	26.1
Tuna, raw					
Albacore	3 oz.	150	6.0	60	36.0
Bluefin	3 oz.	122	4.2	32	30.9
■ Yellowfin	3 oz.	92	0.8	38	7.8
Tuna, canned					
Light, in oil, drained	3 oz.	225	19.1	36	76.0
■ Light, in water, drained	3 oz.	90	1.5	36	15.0
White, in oil, drained	3 oz.	210	15.0	36	64.0
■ White, in water, drained	3 oz.	90	1.0	36	10.0
Turbot, raw	3 oz.	81	2.5	41	27.7
Whitefish					
Raw	3 oz.	114	5.0	51	39.4
Smoked	3½ oz.	160	7.0	54	39.0
■Whiting					
Raw	3 oz.	77	1.1	57	12.8
Cooked	3 oz.	98	1.4	71	12.8
Yellowtail, raw	3 oz.	124	4.5	38	32.6

FLOUR & BAKING INGREDIENTS

Item	PORTION	CALORIES	FAT GRAMS	CHOLESTEROL	% OF FAT
Almond paste, packed	1 tb.	63	3.9	0	55.7
Bisquick, mix, General Mills	1 cup	480	16	0	30.0
Butterscotch baking chips	1 oz.	?	8.0	?	?
Carob chips, nuggets	1 cup	140	7.0	0	45.0
Chocolate					
Bitter or baking	1 oz.	143	15.0	0	94.4
Sweet German, Bakers	1 oz.	142	9.4	0	59.5

Item	PORTION	CAL-ORIES	FAT GRAMS	CHOLES-TEROL	% OF FAT
Chocolate chips					
Bakers	1 oz.	129	5.6	0	39.0
Milk, Hershey	1 oz.	150	7.9	0	47.4
Chocolate morsels, Nestle's	1 oz.	149	8.9	0	53.7
Cocoa powder, low- or medium-fat, dry	1 oz.	62	3.6	0	52.2
■Cornmeal					
Degermed, yellow	1 cup	505	2.3	0	4.0
Yellow, enriched, Quaker	1 cup	544	2.4	0	3.9
Flour					
■ Bread	1 cup	495	2.3	0	4.1
Buckwheat, dark	1 cup	326	2.4	0	6.6
■ Cake	1 cup	395	0.9	0	2.0
■ Carob	1 cup	185	0.7	0	3.4
■ Corn, whole grain	1 cup	422	4.5	0	9.5
Oat blend					
Raw	1 cup	229	6.5	0	25.5
■ Gold, yellow	1 cup	390	3.0	0	6.9
Potato	1 cup	400	0.8	0	1.8
■ Rye, medium	1 cup	361	1.8	0	4.4
Soybean, full fat	1 cup	371	17.6	0	42.7
■ Wheat, self-rising	1 cup	443	1.2	0	2.4
■ White	1 cup	455	1.2	0	2.3
■ Whole Wheat	1 cup	407	2.2	0	4.8
Graham cracker crumbs	1 oz.	109	2.6	0	21.4
Honey	1 cup	86	2.6	0	21.4
■Molasses, cane	1 cup	66	0.0	0	0.0
■Sugar					
Brown	1 cup	106	0.0	0	0.0
Granulated, white	1 cup	109	0.0	0	0.0
Powdered	1 cup	109	0.0	0	0.0
■Syrup, cane	1 cup	75	0.0	0	0.0
Yeast, active, dry	1 pkg.	80	0.5	0	5.6

■ Contains less than 20% fat   88

Item	PORTION	CAL-ORIES	FAT GRAMS	CHOLES-TEROL	% OF FAT
Yeast extract, Marmite	1 tb.	32	0.0	0	0.0

FROZEN FOODS

Beef
Burrito

Item	PORTION	CAL-ORIES	FAT GRAMS	CHOLES-TEROL	% OF FAT
Little Juan					
w/bean, spicy	10 oz.	814	39.2	–	43.3
w/potato	5 oz.	389	16.5	–	38.2
Patio, w/bean & red chili peppers	5 oz.	340	13.0	–	34.4
Weight Watchers, beefsteak	7.6 oz.	310	12.0	70	34.8
Chipped, creamed					
Banquet	4 oz.	100	4.0	–	36.0
Stouffer's	11 oz.	460	32.0	–	62.6
Chimichanga					
Marquez, shredded	5 oz.	351	17.0	–	43.6
Old El Paso					
Dinner	11 oz.	540	21.0	–	35.0
Entree	1 piece	380	23.0	–	54.5
Chopped dinner, Banquet	11 oz.	420	32.0	80	68.6
Chopped sirloin					
Le Menu	11½ oz.	400	18.0	–	40.5
Swanson, 4-compartment	10¾ oz.	340	16.0	–	42.3
Chopped steak, Swanson Hungry Man dinner	16¾ oz.	640	37.0	–	52.0
Dijon, w/pasta & vegetables, Stouffer's Right Course	9½ oz.	290	9.0	40	27.9
Enchilada					
Banquet, dinner	12 oz.	500	15.0	–	27.0

■ Contains less than 20% fat

Item	PORTION	CAL-ORIES	FAT GRAMS	CHOLES-TEROL	% OF FAT
■ Healthy Choice	13.4 oz.	370	5.0	–	12.2
Old El Paso, entree	1 piece	210	13.0	10	55.7
Patio, dinner	13¼ oz.	520	24.0	40	41.5
Weight Watchers	9.1 oz.	300	13.0	45	39.0
Fajita					
■ Healthy Choice	7 oz.	210	4.0	35	17.1
Weight Watchers	6¾ oz.	250	7.0	30	25.2
■London broil	7.4 oz.	140	3.0	40	19.3
w/mushroom					
sauce, Weight					
Watchers					
Meatloaf dinner					
Armour Dinner	11¼ oz.	360	17.0	65	42.5
Classics					
Banquet	11 oz.	440	27.0	5	55.2
Banquet, Healthy	11 oz.	270	7.0	30	23.0
Balance					
Morton	10 oz.	310	17.0	50	31.9
Oriental style,	8⅝ oz.	250	7.0	40	25.2
Stouffer's Lean					
Cuisine					
Pepper steak					
Armour Classics	9 oz.	260	6.0	40	20.8
Dining Lite					
■ Chun King	13 oz.	310	3.0	–	8.7
■ Healthy Choice	1 dinner	260	4.9	–	17.0
dinner					
La Choy	10 oz.	280	8.0	36	25.7
Stouffer's	10½ oz.	330	11.0	–	30.0
■ Ultra Slim Fast,	12 oz.	270	4.0	–	13.3
w/parsley rice					
Pot pie					
Banquet	7 oz.	510	33.0	25	58.2
Empire Kosher	8 oz.	540	30.0	–	50.0
Swanson Hungry	16 oz.	610	31.0	–	45.7
Man					

■ Contains less than 20% fat   90

Item	PORTION	CAL- ORIES	FAT GRAMS	CHOLES- TEROL	% OF FAT
Pot Roast					
Budget Gourmet, Light & Healthy	1 dinner	230	7.0	60	27.1
■ Healthy Choice	11 oz.	260	4.0	45	13.8
Le Menu	10 oz.	330	13.0	–	35.4
Stouffer's Right Course	9¼ oz.	220	7.0	35	28.6
Ragout w/rice pilaf, Stouffer's Right Course	10 oz.	300	8.0	50	24.0
Salisbury steak					
Budget Gourmet, Light & Healthy	1 dinner	220	6.0	25	24.5
Armour Classics Dining Lite	9 oz.	200	8.0	55	36.0
Healthy Choice	11½ oz.	300	7.0	50	21.0
Le Menu					
Regular	10½ oz.	370	20.0	–	48.6
■ Healthy style	1 dinner	270	5.1	–	17.0
Stouffer's Lean Cuisine	9½ oz.	280	15.0	100	48.2
Swanson Hungry Man Dinner	16½ oz.	680	41.0	–	54.3
Weight Watchers, Romana	8¾ oz.	310	13.0	80	37.7
Short ribs, boneless					
Armour Dinner Classics	9¾ oz.	380	16.0	90	37.9
Stouffer's, w/gravy	9 oz.	350	20.0	–	51.4
■Sirloin roast, Armour Dinner Classics	10.4 oz.	190	4.0	55	18.9
Sirloin tips					
Healthy Choice	11¾ oz.	270	6.9	–	22.9
Le Menu dinner	11½ oz.	400	18.0	–	40.5
Swanson home- style recipe	7 oz.	160	5.0	–	28.2

Item	PORTION	CAL-ORIES	FAT GRAMS	CHOLES-TEROL	% OF FAT
Ultra Slim Fast vegetable & beef tips	12 oz.	210	5.0	50	21.5
Weight Watchers w/mushrooms in wine sauce	7½ oz.	250	8.0	85	25.2
Sliced					
Morton dinner	10 oz.	220	5.0	65	20.4
Swanson Hungry Man dinner	15¼ oz.	450	12.0	–	24.0
Steak Diane, Armour Classic Lite	10 oz.	290	9.0	80	27.9
Stew, Banquet Family Entree	7 oz.	140	5.0	–	32.1
Stroganoff					
Budget Gourmet Light entree	8¾ oz.	290	12.0	–	37.2
Le Menu dinner	10 oz.	430	24.0	–	50.2
Weight Watchers	9 oz.	320	13.0	70	36.6
Swiss steak, 4-compartment dinner, Swanson	10 oz.	350	11.0	–	28.3
Szechuan style					
■ Chun King	13 oz.	340	3.0	–	8.0
Stouffer's Lean Cuisine w/noodles & vegetables	9¼ oz.	260	10.0	100	34.6
■Teriyaki, Armour Dining Lite	9 oz.	270	5.0	45	16.7
Cheese					
Enchilada					
Banquet, dinner	12 oz.	550	19.0	–	31.1
Old El Paso entree	1 serv.	250	12.0	–	43.2
Weight Watchers, ranchero	8.9 oz.	360	18.0	60	45.0

■ Contains less than 20% fat

Item	PORTION	CAL-ORIES	FAT GRAMS	CHOLES-TEROL	% OF FAT
Chicken					
A la king					
Armour Classics Lite	11¼ oz.	290	7.0	55	21.7
Le Menu dinner	10¼ oz.	330	13.0	–	35.4
Weight Watchers	9 oz.	240	6.0	20	28.0
■A L'orange, Healthy Choice	9½ oz.	260	2.0	45	6.9
Au gratin, Budget Gourmet Light entree	9.1 oz.	250	11.0	–	39.6
BBQ Breast fillet, Tyson	3 oz.	110	3.0	35	24.5
■Burgundy dinner, Armour Classics Light	10 oz.	210	2.0	45	8.6
Burrito, Weight Watchers	7.6 oz.	310	13.0	60	37.7
Cacciatore					
Healthy Choice	12.5 oz.	310	3.0	35	9.0
Lean Cuisine, w/vermicelli	10.8 oz.	280	7.0	45	22.5
Stouffer's Lean Cuisine, w/vermicelli	10⅞ oz.	250	7.0	45	25.2
Swanson Home-style	10.9 oz.	260	8.0	–	27.7
■Chow mein					
Armour Classics, w/rice	9 oz.	180	2.0	30	10.0
Chun King	13 oz.	370	6.0	85	14.6
Healthy Choice	8½ oz.	220	3.0	45	12.3
■ Lean Cuisine, w/rice	9 oz.	240	5.0	30	18.7
Stouffer's Lean Cuisine	11¼ oz.	250	5.0	35	18.0
■ Ultra Slim Fast	12 oz.	320	6.0	60	16.9

Item	PORTION	CAL-ORIES	FAT GRAMS	CHOLES-TEROL	% OF FAT
Cordon bleu dinner, Le Menu	11 oz.	460	20.0	–	39.1
Creamed, Stouffer's	6½ oz.	300	21.0	–	63.0
Dijon entree, Le Menu, healthy style	8 oz.	240	7.0	40	26.2
Divan, Stouffer's	8½ oz.	320	20.0	–	56.2
Enchilada					
■ Healthy Balance	11 oz.	300	4.0	–	12.0
■ Healthy Choice	13.4 oz.	340	5.0	–	13.2
Old El Paso					
Dinner, festive	11 oz.	460	18.0	–	35.2
Entree w/sour cream sauce	1 serv.	280	19.0	–	61.1
Weight Watchers Suiza	9.4 oz.	330	15.0	50	40.9
Fajita					
■ Healthy Choice	7 oz.	200	3.0	35	13.5
Weight Watchers	6¾ oz.	210	5.0	30	21.4
Fettucini, Weight Watchers	8¼ oz.	290	10.0	35	31.0
■Fiesta Chicken, Smart Ones, Weight Watchers	8 oz.	210	1.0	20	4.3
Francais, Tyson	9½ oz.	280	14.0	–	45.0
Fried					
Banquet					
Assorted pieces	32 oz.	1650	95.0	–	51.8
Breast portion	11½ oz.	440	22.0	–	45.0
Thigh & drum-stick	12½ oz.	500	28.0	–	50.4
Country Pride, chunks	12 oz.	1104	80.0	–	65.2
Swanson					
Assorted, pre-fried	3¼ oz.	270	16.0	–	53.3
Nibbles	3¼ oz.	300	19.0	–	57.0

■ Contains less than 20% fat

Item	PORTION	CAL-ORIES	FAT GRAMS	CHOLES-TEROL	% OF FAT
Fried meal					
Banquet dinner	10 oz.	400	22.0	–	49.5
Kid Cuisine	7¼ oz.	420	22.0	–	47.1
Swanson					
4-compartment dinner					
BBQ flavor	10 oz.	540	22.0	–	36.7
White meat	10¼ oz.	550	25.0	–	40.9
Homestyle Recipe	7 oz.	390	21.0	–	48.5
Weight Watchers, patty	6½ oz.	340	16.0	50	42.3
Glazed					
Armour Dinner Classics	10¾ oz.	300	16.0	60	48.0
■ Healthy Choice	8½ oz.	230	3.0	50	11.7
Stouffer's Lean Cuisine w/vegetable rice	8½ oz.	270	8.0	55	26.7
■Herb roasted, Healthy Choice	11 oz.	260	3.0	40	10.4
Kiev, Tyson	9¼ oz.	520	33.0	–	57.1
■Lemon Herb Chicken Piccata, Smart Ones, Weight Watchers	7.5 oz.	160	0.9	5	5.0
Lemon pepper breast, Tyson	2.75 oz.	110	3.0	35	24.5
Mandarin, Budget Gourmet, w/rice	10 oz.	300	7.0	40	21.0
■Marinara, Tyson Healthy Portion	13¾ oz.	330	7.0	–	19.1
Marsala, breast, w/vegetables, Stouffer's Lean Cuisine	8⅛ oz.	190	5.0	80	23.7

■ Contains less than 20% fat

Item	PORTION	CAL-ORIES	FAT GRAMS	CHOLES-TEROL	% OF FAT
Mesquite					
Armour Dinner Classics	9½ oz.	370	16.0	55	38.1
■ Healthy Choice	10½ oz.	310	2.0	45	5.8
■ Tyson Healthy Portion	13¼ oz.	330	5.0	–	13.6
■ Ultra Slim Fast	12 oz.	440	1.0	45	20.0
■Oriental, Healthy Choice	11¼ oz.	230	1.0	35	3.9
Oriental breast strips, Tyson	2.75 oz.	110	3.0	40	24.5
Parmigiana					
Armour Dinner Classics	11½ oz.	370	19.0	75	46.2
Budget Gourmet Light & Hearty	11 oz.	260	8.0	–	27.7
Celentano	9 oz.	400	21.0	87	47.2
■ Healthy Choice	11½ oz.	280	3.0	60	9.6
Stouffer's Lean Cuisine	10 oz.	260	8.0	80	27.7
Pot Pie					
Banquet	7 oz.	550	36.0	35	58.9
Empire Kosher	8 oz.	463	21.0	–	40.8
Stouffer's	10 oz.	530	33.0	–	56.0
■ Swanson Hungry Man	16 oz.	630	35.0	–	19.7
■Salsa, Healthy Choice	11¼ oz.	240	2.0	–	7.5
■Sesame, Tyson, Healthy Portion	13½ oz.	390	5.0	–	11.5
■Southwestern style, Healthy Choice	12½ oz.	340	5.0	–	13.2
Sweet & Sour					
■ Armour Classics Lite	11 oz.	240	2.0	35	7.5
Banquet, Healthy Balance	10 oz.	260	6.0	45	20.8

■ Contains less than 20% fat

Item	PORTION	CAL-ORIES	FAT GRAMS	CHOLES-TEROL	% OF FAT
Budget Gourmet w/rice	10 oz.	340	5.0	30	39.7
■ Healthy Choice	11½ oz.	280	2.0	50	6.4
■ La Choy fresh & lite	10 oz.	260	3.0	53	10.4
■ Ultra Slim Fast	12 oz.	330	2.0	–	5.4
Tyson	11 oz.	420	15.0	–	32.1
■ Weight Watchers tenders	10.2 oz.	240	1.0	40	3.7
Tenderloins, Stouffer's Right Course, in peanut sauce w/linguini & vegetables	9¼ oz.	330	10.0	50	27.3
■Walnut, crunchy, Chun King	13 oz.	310	5.0	–	14.5

Pasta & Pizza
Agnoletti entree, Buitoni

Item	PORTION	CAL-ORIES	FAT GRAMS	CHOLES-TEROL	% OF FAT
■ Cheese filled	2 oz.	196	3.3	–	15.1
Meat filled	2 oz.	206	4.8	–	21.0
■Angel hair pasta, Smart Ones, Weight Watchers	8.5 oz.	120	1.0	0	7.5

Cannelloni
  Cheese

Item	PORTION	CAL-ORIES	FAT GRAMS	CHOLES-TEROL	% OF FAT
Armour Dining Lite	9 oz.	310	9.0	70	26.1
Stouffer's Lean Cuisine	9⅛ oz.	260	10.0	35	34.6
Beef & pork w/mornay sauce, Stouffer's Lean Cuisine	9⅝ oz.	260	10.0	45	34.6

Item	PORTION	CAL-ORIES	FAT GRAMS	CHOLES-TEROL	% OF FAT
Fettucini Alfredo					
■ Healthy Choice	8 oz.	270	6.0	45	20.0
Stouffer's	10 oz.	540	38.0	–	63.3
Fettucini primavera, Green Giant	9½ oz.	230	8.0	25	31.3
Lasagna al forno, Buitoni	8 oz.	327	13.6	–	37.4
Lasagna, cheese					
Armour Dining Lite	9 oz.	260	6.0	30	20.8
Celentano	10 oz.	460	24.0	92	47.0
Stouffer's	10½ oz.	360	13.0	–	32.5
Weight Watchers, Italian cheese	11 oz.	290	7.0	–	21.7
Lasagna, garden vegetable, Le Menu healthy style	10½ oz.	260	8.0	25	27.7
Lasagna w/meat sauce					
Armour Dining Lite	9 oz.	260	6.0	40	20.8
Buitoni	5 oz.	212	8.3	–	35.2
■ Healthy Choice	9 oz.	260	5.0	20	17.3
Stouffer's Lean Cuisine	10¼ oz.	270	8.0	60	26.7
Lasagna primavera, Celentano	11 oz.	330	14.0	90	38.2
Lasagna, seafood, light, Mrs. Paul's	9½ oz.	290	8.0	57	24.8
Lasagna, tuna, w/spinach noodles & vegetables, Stouffer's Lean Cuisine	9¾ oz.	270	10.0	35	33.3
Lasagne w/vegetables and tofu, Legume	12 oz.	240	8.0	0	30.0

Item	PORTION	CAL- ORIES	FAT GRAMS	CHOLES- TEROL	% OF FAT
Lasagna, zucchini, Stouffer's Lean Cuisine	11 oz.	260	7.0	25	24.2
Linguini w/clam sauce, Stouffer's Lean Cuisine	9⅝ oz.	270	7.0	30	23.3
Linguini, seafood, Weight Watch- ers	9 oz.	210	7.0	5	30.0
■Linguini w/shrimp, Healthy Choice	9½ oz.	230	2.0	55	7.8
Macaroni & beef, w/tomatoes, Stouffer's	11½ oz.	340	14.0	–	37.1
Macaroni & cheese					
Banquet dinner	10 oz.	420	20.0	30	42.9
Birds Eye Classics	10 oz.	472	22.0	66	41.9
Stouffer's	12 oz.	500	26.0	–	46.8
Macaroni & cheese pot pie, Swanson	7 oz.	200	8.0	–	36.0
Manicotti					
Buitoni, plain	5½ oz.	310	15.0	–	43.5
Celentano	10 oz.	380	14.0	82	33.2
Florentine, Legume	11 oz.	260	7.0	0	22.0
Stouffer's	8 oz.	234	10.9	34	4.7
Weight Watchers, in tomato sauce	9¼ oz.	300	13.0	90	39.0
Noodles Romanoff, Stouffer's	8 oz.	347	19.1	39	49.5
Pasta meal					
■ Alfredo sauce, Ul- tra Slim Fast	½ cup	120	2.0	–	15.0
■ Cheese sauce, Ultra Slim Fast	½ cup	115	2.0	–	15.5
Dijon, Green Giant	9½ oz.	260	17.0	55	58.8
Florentine	9½ oz.	230	9.0	25	35.2

■ Contains less than 20% fat

Item	PORTION	CAL-ORIES	FAT GRAMS	CHOLES-TEROL	% OF FAT
Marinara					
■ Birds Eye Classics	10 oz.	230	4.0	2	15.6
Green Giant	6 oz.	180	5.0	0	25.0
■ Ultra Slim Fast, w/vegetables	12 oz.	290	3.0	–	9.3
Primavera					
Weight Watchers	8½ oz.	260	11.0	5	38.1
■ Tomato and herb sauce, Ultra Slim Fast	½ cup	110	1.5	–	12.5
Pizza, bacon, Totino's	10 oz.	740	40.0	–	48.6
Pizza, Canadian style bacon					
Jeno's	7.7 oz.	240	10.0	–	37.5
Stouffer's French bread	11⅝ oz.	720	28.0	–	35.0
Pizza, cheese					
Banquet Zap, French bread	4½ oz.	310	10.0	35	29.0
■ Healthy Choice, French bread	5.6 oz.	300	3.0	–	9.0
Jeno's 4-pack	8.9 oz.	640	32.0	–	45.0
■ Kid Cuisine	6½ oz.	240	4.0	20	15.0
■ McCain Ellio's Healthy slices	5 oz.	320	4.0	–	11.2
Pepperidge Farm, croissant crust	1	430	23.0	–	48.1
Stouffer's, French bread	½ pkg.	340	13.0	–	34.4
Totino's, three cheese	¼ of pie	490	25.0	65	45.9
Weight Watchers, regular	5¾ oz.	310	8.0	40	23.2
Pizza, combination					
Pappalo's, thin crust	⅙ of pie	260	10.0	–	34.6

Item	PORTION	CAL-ORIES	FAT GRAMS	CHOLES-TEROL	% OF FAT
Weight Watchers, deluxe	6¾ oz.	300	8.0	7	24.0
Pizza, deluxe, Weight Watchers, French bread	6.1 oz.	310	13.0	10	37.7
Pizza, English muffin, Empire Kosher	2 oz.	140	4.0	–	25.7
Pizza, hamburger, Fox Deluxe	½ of pie	260	12.0	–	41.5
Pizza, pepperoni					
Banquet Zap, French bread	4½ oz.	350	16.0	40	41.1
Pappalo's, pan style	4.2 oz.	330	14.0	–	38.2
Weight Watchers, regular	5.9 oz.	320	9.0	45	25.3
Pizza, sausage					
Jeno's, 4-pack	2.4 oz.	180	9.0	–	45.0
Pappalo's, thin crust	3.7 oz.	250	9.0	–	32.4
Stouffer's, French bread					
Regular	6 oz.	420	20.0	–	42.8
Lean Cuisine	6 oz.	350	11.0	45	28.3
Weight Watchers	6¼ oz.	310	8.0	45	26.4
Pizza, Suprema, Celeste	9 oz.	678	39.2	–	52.0
Pizza, vegetable					
Wolfgang Puck	2.7 oz.	140	4.0	5	25.7
Stouffer's, French bread	6.4 oz.	420	20.0	–	42.9
Tombstone Light	½ pizza	170	5.0	5	27.6
Ravioli, cheese					
■ Healthy Choice, baked	9 oz.	250	2.0	–	7.2
Weight Watchers, baked	9 oz.	240	6.0	–	22.5

■ Contains less than 20% fat

Item	PORTION	CAL-ORIES	FAT GRAMS	CHOLES-TEROL	% OF FAT
Spaghetti, w/beef, Armour Dining Lite	9 oz.	220	8.0	20	32.7
Spaghetti w/meatballs					
Banquet dinner	10 oz.	290	10.0	30	31.0
■ Morton dinner	10 oz.	200	3.0	10	13.5
Stouffer's	12⅞ oz.	370	11.0	–	26.7
Spaghetti w/meat sauce					
Banquet casserole	8 oz.	270	8.0	–	26.7
■ Healthy Choice	10 oz.	280	6.0	20	19.3
Kid Cuisine	9¼ oz.	310	12.0	35	34.8
Weight Watchers	10½ oz.	280	7.0	35	22.5
Tortellini, cheese					
Green Giant, marinara	5½ oz.	260	9.0	–	31.1
Stouffer's, w/Alfredo sauce	8⅞ oz.	600	40.0	–	60.0
Seafood					
Clam					
Gorton strips, crunchy	3½ oz.	330	22.0	30	60.0
Mrs. Paul's, fried, light	2½ oz.	200	9.0	15	40.5
Cod fillet					
■ Captain's Choice	3 oz.	89	1.0	47	10.1
■ Gorton's Fishmarket Fresh	5 oz.	110	1.0	–	8.2
Mrs. Paul's, light	1 piece	240	11.0	50	41.2
Fish cake					
Captain's Choice	1	130	6.0	–	41.5
Mrs. Paul's	1	95	3.5	10	33.1
Fish & chips, Swanson Homestyle Recipe	6½ oz.	340	16.0	–	42.3

■ Contains less than 20% fat

Item	PORTION	CAL-ORIES	FAT GRAMS	CHOLES-TEROL	% OF FAT
Fish dinner					
Morton	9¾ oz.	370	13.0	65	31.6
Weight Watchers, oven fried	7.1 oz.	300	13.0	15	39.0
Fish fillet					
Almondine, Gorton's	1 pkg.	340	25.0	100	66.2
Au gratin, Weight Watchers	9¼ oz.	200	6.0	60	27.0
Batter dipped, Mrs. Paul's	1	165	8.5	30	46.4
■ Breaded, Healthy Treasures, Mrs. Paul's	1	170	3.0	25	16.5
Dijon, Mrs. Paul's light entree	8¾ oz.	200	14.0	60	63.0
Divan, Stouffer's Lean Cuisine	12⅜ oz.	260	7.0	85	24.2
Light, in butter sauce, Mrs. Paul's	1 pc.	70	3.0	20	38.6
Mornay, Mrs. Paul's	9 oz.	230	10.0	80	39.1
Fish sticks					
Captain's Choice	1	76	3.0	31	35.5
Gorton's potato crisp	1	65	4.0	6	80.0
Mrs. Paul's					
Battered	1	52	3.0	6	51.9
Breaded, crispy, crunchy	1	35	1.5	5	38.6
Florentine, Mrs. Paul's	8 oz.	220	8.0	95	33.0
■Flounder fillet, plain, Captain's Choice	3 oz.	99	1.0	58	9.1

Item	PORTION	CAL-ORIES	FAT GRAMS	CHOLES-TEROL	% OF FAT
Flounder fillet, stuffed, Gorton's	1 pkg.	350	18.0	120	46.3
Haddock, crunchy batter, fillet, Mrs. Paul's	1	95	2.5	12	23.7
Haddock in lemon butter, Gorton's	1 pkg.	360	1.0	100	52.5
■Halibut steak, Captain's Choice	3 oz.	119	2.0	35	15.1
Lobster newburg, Stouffer's	6½ oz.	380	32.0	–	75.8
■Shrimp chow mein dinner, La Choy	12 oz.	220	1.0	–	4.1
■Shrimp creole					
Armour Classics Lite	11¼ oz.	260	2.0	45	6.9
Healthy Choice	11¼ oz.	210	1.0	65	4.3
Shrimp w/lobster sauce, La Choy, fresh & lite	10 oz.	240	6.2	118	23.2
■Shrimp marinara, Healthy Choice	10½ oz.	220	1.0	50	4.1
Shrimp, marinated in batter, Gorton's	2.7 oz.	170	9.0	55	47.6
Shrimp scampi, Gorton's	1 pkg.	470	32.0	130	61.3
■Shrimp, stir fry, Chef's Choice	¾ cup	101	0.09	47	1.0
■Sole au gratin dinner, Healthy Choice	11 oz.	270	5.0	55	16.7
Sole w/lemon butter sauce, Gorton's	1 pkg.	180	8.0	90	40.0
Sole, stuffed w/newburg sauce, Weight Watchers	10½ oz.	310	9.0	5	26.1

■ Contains less than 20% fat

Item	PORTION	CAL-ORIES	FAT GRAMS	CHOLES-TEROL	% OF FAT
Turkey					
■Breast of, Healthy Choice	10½ oz.	290	5.0	45	15.5
Dijon, Stouffer's Lean Cuisine	9½ oz.	270	10.0	60	33.3
Dinner					
Banquet	10½ oz.	390	20.0	40	46.1
Morton	10 oz.	226	6.0	45	23.9
Swanson 4-compartment	11½ oz.	350	11.0	–	28.3
Divan, Le Menu Healthy Style	10 oz.	260	7.0	60	24.2
Glazed, Le Menu Healthy Style entree	8¼ oz.	260	6.0	35	20.8
Pot Pie					
Banquet	7 oz.	510	31.0	40	54.7
Morton	7 oz.	420	28.0	40	60.0
Swanson	8 oz.	430	24.0	–	50.2
Regular	7 oz.	380	21.0	–	49.7
Hungry Man	16 oz.	650	36.0	–	49.8
Sliced					
w/mushroom gravy, Le Menu	10½ oz.	300	7.0	–	21.0
in mushroom sauce, Stouffer's Lean Cuisine	8 oz.	240	7.0	50	26.2
w/dressing & gravy, Armour Dinner Classics	11½ oz.	320	12.0	50	33.7
Stuffed breast, Weight Watchers	8½ oz.	260	10.0	80	34.6
Tetrazzini, Stouffer's	10 oz.	380	20.0	–	47.4

Item	PORTION	CAL-ORIES	FAT GRAMS	CHOLES-TEROL	% OF FAT
Veal					
Parmigiana					
Armour Dinner Classics	11¼ oz.	400	22.0	55	49.5
Le Menu	11½ oz.	390	17.0	–	39.2
Morton	10 oz.	260	8.0	35	27.7
Weight Watchers patty	8.4 oz.	220	10.0	65	40.9
Vegetable					
Eggplant					
Parmigiana					
Buitoni	5 oz.	168	8.7	–	44.8
Celentano	10-oz.	350	19.0	40	48.9
Mrs. Paul's	5 oz.	240	16.0	15	60.0
Rollatines Celentano	11 oz.	320	14.0	122	39.4
Potatoes					
■ Baked, w/broccoli & cheese sauce, Healthy Choice	10 oz.	240	5.0	15	19.0
■ Country Style Dinner Fries, Ore-Ida	3 oz.	110	2.0	0	16.5
■ Lite Crinkle cuts, Ore-Ida	3 oz.	90	2.0	0	20.0
■ Whole, small, Ore-Ida	3 oz.	70	0.0	0	0.0
■Stir fry					
Flav-R-Pac, w/rice	1 cup	80	0.0	0	0.0
Shanghai, oriental	5.3 oz.	75	1.0	0	12.0

■ Contains less than 20% fat   106

Item	PORTION	CAL-ORIES	FAT GRAMS	CHOLES-TEROL	% OF FAT

FRUITS†

Item	PORTION	CAL-ORIES	FAT GRAMS	CHOLES-TEROL	% OF FAT
■Apples					
Fresh	1	81	0.0	0	0.0
Dried	1	19	0.0	0	0.0
■ Dried, chips, Weight Watchers	¾ oz.	70	0.0	0	0.0
■Applesauce					
Canned, unsweetened	½ cup	52	0.0	0	0.0
Canned, sweetened	½ cup	97	0.0	0	0.0
■Apricots					
Fresh	1	18	0.0	0	0.0
Canned, w/skin, heavy syrup	½ cup	114	0.0	0	0.0
Dried, uncooked	1	17	0.0	0	0.0
Avocado, fresh					
California	1	306	29.8	0	87.6
Florida	1	339	26.7	0	70.8
■Banana, fresh	1	109	0.0	0	0.0
■Blackberries					
Fresh	½ cup	37	0.0	0	0.0
Frozen, unsweetened, not thawed	½ cup	48	0.0	0	0.0
■Blueberries					
Fresh	½ cup	41	0.0	0	0.0
Frozen, unsweetened	½ cup	42	0.0	0	0.0
■Boysenberries, frozen, unsweetened	½ cup	31	0.0	0	0.0
■Breadfruit, fresh	1	527	1.2	0	2.0

■ Contains less than 20% fat
†There are only traces of fat in all fruits. We have listed the fat only if it is over .5 grams per serving.

Item	PORTION	CALORIES	FAT GRAMS	CHOLESTEROL	% OF FAT
■Cantaloupe, fresh	¼	45	0.0	0	0.0
■Casaba, fresh	⅛	53	0.0	0	0.0
■Cherries, fresh					
Sour, red w/o pits	½ cup	39	0.0	0	0.0
Sweet	½ cup	52	0.0	0	0.0
■Cherries, canned					
Sour, red, water-packed	½ cup	44	0.0	0	0.0
Sour, red, heavy syrup	½ cup	127	0.0	0	0.0
Sweet, water-packed	½ cup	62	0.0	0	0.0
Sweet, heavy syrup	½ cup	107	0.2	0	1.7
■Cherries, Maraschino	½ cup	162	0.0	0	0.0
Coconut					
Fresh	1 whole	1,349	127.7	0	85.2
Shredded, dried, sweetened	1½ cup	232	16.4	0	63.6
■Crab apples, fresh	1 each	23	0.0	0	0.0
■Cranberries, fresh	½ cup	23	0.0	0	0.0
■Cranberries, dried	½ cup	416	1.9	0	4.0
■Cranberry sauce, canned, sweetened	½ cup	209	0.0	0	0.0
■Cranberry/orange relish	½ cup	245	0.0	0	0.0
■Currants, fresh					
Black, European	½ cup	35	0.0	0	0.0
Red or white	½ cup	31	0.0	0	0.0
■Dates, domestic	1	23	0.0	0	0.0
■Figs					
Fresh, medium	1	37	0.0	0	0.0
Dried	1	48	0.0	0	0.0
Canned, light syrup	½ cup	87	0.0	0	0.0
■Fruit cocktail, canned					
Juice-packed	½ cup	57	0.0	0	0.0
In heavy syrup	½ cup	93	0.0	0	0.0

■ Contains less than 20% fat

Item	PORTION	CAL-ORIES	FAT GRAMS	CHOLES-TEROL	% OF FAT
■Fruit salad, canned					
Water-packed	½ cup	37	0.0	0	0.0
In heavy syrup	½ cup	93	0.0	0	0.0
■Gooseberries					
Fresh	½ cup	33	0.0	0	0.0
Canned, in heavy syrup	½ cup	114	0.0	0	0.0
■Grapefruit					
Fresh	1	77	0.0	0	0.0
Canned, sweetened	½ cup	76	0.0	0	0.0
■Grapes, fresh					
Concord	½ cup	29	0.0	0	0.0
Emperor	½ cup	57	0.0	0	0.0
Thompson	½ cup	57	0.0	0	0.0
■Guavas, common, fresh	1	41	0.0	0	0.0
■Honeydew, fresh, cubed	½ cup	30	0	0	0.0
■Kiwi fruit	1	44	0.0	0	0.0
■Kumquat, fresh	1	12	0.0	0	0.0
■Lemons, fresh					
With peel	1	22	0.0	0	0.0
Without peel	1	16	0.0	0	0.0
■Lemon Juice					
Fresh	½ cup	31	0.0	0	0.0
Canned or bottled, unsweetened	½ cup	26	0.0	0	0.0
■Limes, fresh	1	20	0.0	0	0.0
■Lime juice					
Fresh	½ cup	33	0.0	0	0.0
Canned or bottled, unsweetened	½ cup	26	0.0	0	0.0
■Loganberries, fresh	½ cup	45	0.0	0	0.0
■Mangoes, fresh	1	133	0.0	0	0.0
■Mixed fruit					
Chunky, lite, canned, Libby's	½ cup	54	0.0	0	0.0

■ Contains less than 20% fat   109

Item	PORTION	CAL-ORIES	FAT GRAMS	CHOLES-TEROL	% OF FAT
Dried	½ cup	69	0.0	0	0.0
Frozen, sweetened	½ cup	123	0.0	0	0.0
■Mulberries, fresh	1	1	0.0	0	0.0
■Nectarines, fresh	1	67	0.0	0	0.0
■Oranges, fresh					
California, navel, diced	½ cup	48	0.0	0	0.0
California, Valencia, diced	½ cup	51	0.0	0	0.0
■Oranges, canned, mandarin, juice-packed	½ cup	46	0.0	0	0.0
■Papayas, fresh, whole	1	88	0.0	0	0.0
■Passion fruit, purple, fresh	1	17	0.0	0	0.0
■Peaches					
Fresh	1	37	0.0	0	0.0
Canned, water-packed	½ cup	29	0.0	0	0.0
Canned, in light syrup	½ cup	69	0.0	0	0.0
Dried	½ cup	191	0.0	0	0.0
Frozen, sliced, sweetened	½ cup	117	0.0	0	0.0
■Pears					
Fresh	1	97	0.0	0	0.0
Canned, in light syrup	½ cup	71	0.0	0	0.0
Dried	½ cup	236	0.0	0	0.0
■Persimmon, native, fresh	1	31	0.0	0	0.0
■Pineapple					
Fresh, diced	½ cup	38	0.0	0	0.0
Canned, chunks, juice-packed	½ cup	75	0.0	0	0.0
■Plantain, cooked	½ cup	85	0.0	0	0.0

■ Contains less than 20% fat   110

Item	PORTION	CAL-ORIES	FAT GRAMS	CHOLES-TEROL	% OF FAT
■Plums					
Fresh	1	35	0.0	0	0.0
Purple, canned, in heavy syrup	½ cup	115	0.0	0	0.0
■Pomegranate pulp, fresh	1	104	0.0	0	0.0
■Prickly pears, fresh	1	42	0.0	0	0.0
■Prunes					
Dried, uncooked,	1 med.	20	0.0	0	0.0
Cooked, no sugar	½ cup	134	0.0	0	0.0
■Quince, fresh	1	52	0.0	0	0.0
■Raisins					
Black	½ cup	217	0.0	0	0.0
Golden	½ cup	219	0.0	0	0.0
■Raspberries					
Black, fresh	½ cup	33	0.0	0	0.0
Red, fresh	½ cup	30	0.0	0	0.0
Red, frozen, sweet-ened	½ cup	129	0.0	0	0.0
■Rhubarb, cooked, added sugar	½ cup	157	0.0	0	0.0
■Strawberries					
Fresh	1 cup	45	0.0	0	0.0
Frozen, unsweet-ened	1 cup	52	0.0	0	0.0
■Tangerines	1	38	0.0	0	0.0
■Watermelon, fresh, diced	½ cup	26	0.0	0	0.0

ICE CREAM, FROZEN YOGURT & NON-DAIRY FROZEN DESSERTS

Ice Cream					
Almond supreme, Good Humor	4 fl. oz.	350	23.3	0	59.9
Banana crumble, Lu-cerne	4 fl. oz.	140	7.0	25	45.0

■ Contains less than 20% fat   111

Item	PORTION	CALORIES	FAT GRAMS	CHOLESTEROL	% OF FAT
Blackberry pecan, Lucerne	4 fl. oz.	150	7.0	25	42.0
Blueberry & cream, Häagen-Dazs	4 fl. oz.	190	8.0	–	37.9
Bon bon, Carnation	1 piece	34	2.4	–	63.5
Brittle bar, Häagen-Dazs	1 bar	370	25.0	–	60.8
Butter brickle, Snow Star	4 fl. oz.	130	7.0	25	48.5
Butter pecan, Häagen-Dazs	4 fl. oz.	290	17.0	–	52.8
Cake roll	1 slice	159	6.9	52	32.0
Chip candy crunch bar, Good Humor	3-fl.-oz. bar	255	17.9	–	63.2
Chocolate					
Baskin-Robbins	4 fl. oz.	264	12.6	35	42.9
Häagen-Dazs	4 fl. oz.	270	17.0	120	56.7
Chocolate chip					
Baskin-Robbins	4 fl. oz.	260	15.0	40	51.9
Lucerne	4 fl. oz.	150	8.0	–	48.0
Chocolate chip bar, Nestlé	2.4-fl.-oz. bar	220	15.0	–	61.4
Chocolate cup, Breyers	5 oz.	160	8.0	20	45.0
Chocolate, dietetic, Lucerne	4 fl. oz.	130	6.0	20	41.5
Chocolate, deep, Häagen-Dazs	4 fl. oz.	290	14.0	–	43.4
■Chocolate fudge bar, Lucerne	3-fl.-oz. bar	125	2.0	6	14.4
Chocolate marshmallow, Lucerne	4 fl. oz.	140	6.0	–	38.6
Chocolate truffle, gourmet, Lucerne	4 fl. oz.	170	7.0	25	37.0
Coffee, Häagen-Dazs	4 fl. oz.	270	17.0	120	56.7

Item	PORTION	CAL-ORIES	FAT GRAMS	CHOLES-TEROL	% OF FAT
Cookies & cream, Lucerne	4 fl. oz.	180	9.0	30	45.0
Drumstick	1	187	9.9	9	47.6
Egg nog, Lucerne	4 fl. oz.	140	7.0	25	45.0
Eskimo pie, original	3 fl. oz.	180	12.0	–	60.0
■Fat-free, Baskin-Robbins	4 fl. oz.	100	0.0	0	0.0
Fat Frog, Good Humor	3-fl.-oz. pop	154	9.2	0	53.8
French vanilla					
Baskin-Robbins	4 fl. oz.	280	18.0	90	57.9
Lucerne	4 fl. oz.	150	8.0	–	48.0
French vanilla, soft serve	½ cup	189	11.3	77	53.8
■Fudge bar, Good Humor	2½-fl.-oz. bar	127	.6	–	4.2
Halo Bar, Good Humor	2½-fl.-oz. bar	230	13.7	0	53.6
Heavenly hash, Lucerne	4 fl. oz.	150	7.0	25	42.0
Honey vanilla, Häagen-Dazs	4 fl. oz.	250	16.0	–	57.6
Klondike light	2.5-fl.-oz. bar	110	7.0	5	57.3
Light, Baskin-Robbins	4 fl. oz.	130	6.0	11	41.5
Macadamia nut, Häagen-Dazs	4 fl. oz.	330	24.0	–	65.4
Maple nut, Lucerne	4 fl. oz.	150	9.0	–	54.0
Mocha double nut, Häagen-Dazs	4 fl. oz.	290	20.0	–	62.1
Neapolitan, Snow Star	4 fl. oz.	120	6.0	20	45.0
Peach					
Häagen-Dazs	4 fl. oz.	210	14.0	–	60.0
Lucerne	4 fl. oz.	140	7.0	25	45.0

Item	PORTION	CAL-ORIES	FAT GRAMS	CHOLES-TEROL	% OF FAT
Peanut butter sundae, Lucerne	4 fl. oz.	140	7.0	25	45.0
■Praline Dream, Baskin-Robbins, Light	4 fl. oz.	130	6.0	11	4.5
Raspberry cream, Häagen-Dazs	4 fl. oz.	180	7.0	–	35.0
Rocky Road, Baskin-Robbins	4 fl. oz.	300	14.0	32	42.0
Rum raisin, Häagen-Dazs	4 fl. oz.	250	17.0	110	61.2
Sandwich, Lucerne	1	125	6.0	20	43.2
Strawberry					
Borden	4 fl. oz.	130	6.0	–	41.5
Häagen-Dazs	4 fl. oz.	250	15.0	95	54.0
Lucerne Gourmet	4 fl. oz.	140	6.0	20	35.0
Strawberry, vanilla & blueberry, Lucerne	4 fl. oz.	140	7.0	25	45.0
Toasted almond bar, Good Humor	3-fl.-oz. bar	212	11.8	–	50.1
Vanilla					
Baskin-Robbins	4 fl. oz.	235	13.1	50	50.2
Häagen-Dazs	4 fl. oz.	260	17.0	125	58.8
Land O'Lakes	4 fl. oz.	140	7.0	30	45.0
Vanilla bar, chocolate covered					
Good Humor	3-fl.-oz. bar	198	13.7	0	62.3
Häagen-Dazs					
Dark chocolate	3.7-fl.-oz. bar	360	26.0	–	65.0
Milk chocolate	3.5-fl.-oz. bar	320	23.0	–	64.7
Vanilla chocolate cup, Good Humor	6 fl. oz.	201	9.2	–	41.2
Vanilla cup, Good Humor	3 fl. oz.	98	5.1	0	46.8

■ Contains less than 20% fat

Item	PORTION	CAL-ORIES	FAT GRAMS	CHOLES-TEROL	% OF FAT
Vanilla Swiss almond, Häagen-Dazs	4 fl. oz.	290	19.0	–	59.0
Frozen Yogurt (see also Frozen, soft serve, p. 50)					
■Low-fat, Colombo	4 fl. oz.	99	2.0	10	18.1
■Non-fat					
Colombo	4 fl. oz.	95	0.0	0	0.0
TCBY	4 fl. oz.	110	1.0	5	8.2
Regular, TCBY, 4% fat	4 fl. oz.	130	3.0	10	20.8
■Sugar-free, TCBY	4 fl. oz.	80	1.0	5	11.2
Non-Dairy Frozen Desserts					
■American Dream, vanilla	4 fl. oz.	134	1.3	0	8.7
■Simple Pleasures, chocolate	4 fl. oz.	140	1.0	0	6.4
Tofutti					
Cappuccino Drop, hardened	½ cup	229	11.9	0	46.8
Chocolate Supreme, hardened	½ cup	208	12.9	0	55.9
Frozen tofu dessert	½ cup	128	6.4	0	45.7
Regular, soft serve	½ cup	157	8.0	0	45.9
Vanilla Love Drops, hardened	½ cup	219	11.9	0	48.9
Vanilla, soft serve	½ cup	199	10.9	0	49.3
Ices & Ice Milk					
■Caramel nut, Lucerne	½ cup	105	2.0	5	17.1
Chocolate					
Lucerne	½ cup	110	2.0	5	16.4
Weight Watchers Grand Collection	½ cup	110	3.0	10	24.5

Item	PORTION	CAL-ORIES	FAT GRAMS	CHOLES-TEROL	% OF FAT
Chocolate chip					
Lucerne	½ cup	100	2.0	5	18.0
Weight Watchers Grand Collection	½ cup	120	4.0	10	30.0
Chocolate, light, Lucerne	½ cup	120	3.0	–	22.5
Chocolate Non Fat Frozen dessert, Sealtest	½ cup	100	0.0	0	0.0
Fudge marble, Weight Watchers Grand Collection	½ cup	120	4.0	5	30.0
■Strawberry, Lucerne	½ cup	95	2.0	5	18.9
Vanilla					
■ Lucerne	½ cup	100	2.0	5	18.0
■ Weight Watchers Grand Collection	½ cup	100	3.0	10	27.0
Vanilla, hardened	½ cup	92	2.8	9	27.4
■Vanilla, soft	½ cup	112	2.3	7	18.5
Other					
■Chocolate Mousse Bar, Weight Watchers	1	35	1.0	5	12.0
■Chocolate Treat Bar, Weight Watchers	1	100	1.0	0	9.0
Cone, plain, w/o ice cream					
■ Baskin-Robbins					
Sugar	1	60	1.0	0	15.0
Waffle	1	140	2.0	0	12.9
■ Comet, sugar	1	40	0.0	–	0.0
■Fruit bar, cherry, Jell-O	1	41	0.1	0	2.2

■ Contains less than 20% fat

Item	PORTION	CAL-ORIES	FAT GRAMS	CHOLES-TEROL	% OF FAT
Fruit & juice bar					
Dole, piña colada	1 bar	80	2.0	0	22.5
■ Minute Maid, all flavors	1 bar	60	0.0	0	0.0
■ Weight Watchers	1 bar	35	0.0	0	0.0
■Fudgesicle					
Regular	1	70	1.0	–	12.7
Fat-free	1	70	0.0	0	0.0
■Gelatin pop, Jell-O	1.8 fl. oz.	35	0.0	0	0.0
■Popsicle	1	64	0.0	0	0.0
Pudding pop, vanilla, Jell-O	1	71	2.0	1	25.4
■Sherbet or sorbet					
Lime, Lucerne	½ cup	120	2.0	5	15.0
Orange					
Baskin-Robbins	½ cup	158	2.4	–	13.7
Häagen-Dazs	½ cup	113	0.0	–	0.0
Rainbow, Baskin-Robbins	½ cup	160	2.0	6	11.2
Sherbet or sorbet & ice cream					
Key lime & vanilla ice cream, Häagen-Dazs	½ cup	190	7.0	–	33.1
Orange & vanilla ice cream					
Häagen-Dazs	½ cup	190	8.0	–	37.9
Lucerne	½ cup	130	5.0	–	34.6
■Sherbet shake mix, orange, Weight Watchers	1 env.	70	0.0	–	0.0
■Sorbet					
Baskin-Robbins, soft serve	½ cup	100	0.0	0	0.0
Frusen Gladje	½ cup	140	0.0	0	0.0

JAMS & JELLIES

Item	PORTION	CAL-ORIES	FAT GRAMS	CHOLES-TEROL	% OF FAT
■Apple butter, Smucker's	1 tb.	36	0.1	0	2.7
■Fruit spread, St. Dalfour	1 tsp.	14	0.0	0	0.0
■Grape jam, Welch's	1 tb.	52	0.0	0	0.0
■Grape jelly, imitation, Smucker's	1 tb.	6	0.0	0	0.0
■Jam	1 tb.	40	0.0	0	0.0
■Jelly	1 tb.	48	0.0	0	0.0
■Marmalade, orange, low sugar, Smucker's	1 tb.	24	0.0	0	0.0
■Raspberry preserves	1 tb.	54	0.0	0	0.0
■Simply Fruit	1 tsp.	14	0.0	0	0.0
■Strawberry preserves	1 tsp.	54	0.0	0	0.0

MEATS

Beef

Item	PORTION	CAL-ORIES	FAT GRAMS	CHOLES-TEROL	% OF FAT
Brisket, flat, lean, braised,	3 oz.	224	13.5	77	54.2
Chuck					
Arm, lean, braised	3 oz.	196	8.5	86	39.0
Blade, lean, braised	3 oz.	230	13.0	90	50.9
Ground					
Extra-lean, broiled	3-oz. patty	218	13.9	71	57.4
Lean, broiled	3-oz. patty	231	15.7	74	61.2
Healthy Choice	3-oz. patty	98	3.0	41	27.0
Rib eye, lean, broiled	3 oz.	191	9.9	68	46.6
Round					
Bottom, lean, braised	3 oz.	189	8.2	82	39.0
Eye, lean, roasted	3 oz.	156	4.0	77	23.0
Tip, lean, roasted	3 oz.	162	6.4	69	35.5

■ Contains less than 20% fat

Item	PORTION	CAL- ORIES	FAT GRAMS	CHOLES- TEROL	% OF FAT
Top, lean, broiled	3 oz.	162	5.3	71	29.4
Short ribs, lean, braised	3 oz.	251	15.4	79	55.2
Sirloin, lean, broiled	3 oz.	177	7.4	76	37.6
Steak, flank, lean, broiled	3 oz.	207	12.7	60	55.2
Tenderloin, lean, broiled	3 oz.	173	7.9	71	41.1
Beefalo					
Patty, cooked	3 oz.	161	5.4	50	30.2
Game					
Boar, roasted	3 oz.	139	3.75	–	25.5
■Buffalo, roasted	3 oz.	111	1.5	93	12.2
■Rabbit, domestic, stewed	3 oz.	175	7.2	73	37.0
■Rabbit, wild, raw	3 oz.	97	2.0	69	18.6
■Venison, roasted	3 oz.	134	2.7	95	18.1
Ham					
Canned					
Hormel 94% fat free	3 oz.	92	3.0	–	29.3
Oscar Mayer Jubilee	3 oz.	87	2.7	42	28.0
Country style, cured, lean	3 oz.	173	10.9	46	56.7
Fresh					
Raw, lean	3 oz.	117	4.5	52	34.6
Roasted, lean & fat,	3 oz.	233	15.1	81	58.3
Loin, roasted, lean only	3 oz.	204	11.7	77	51.6
Loin, sirloin, raw					
Lean only	3 oz.	128	5.7	54	40.0
Lean & fat	3 oz.	235	19.0	60	72.8

■ Contains less than 20% fat

Item	PORTION	CAL-ORIES	FAT GRAMS	CHOLES-TEROL	% OF FAT
Picnic					
Raw, lean only	3 oz.	117	4.5	52	34.6
Simmered, lean only	3 oz.	188	9.1	82	43.6
Cured, unheated, 70% lean	3 oz.	155	9.0	48	52.2
Lamb					
Chop					
Loin, broiled, lean only	3 oz.	160	6.0	44	34.0
Loin, broiled, lean & fat	3 oz.	305	25.0	85	74.0
Rib					
Cooked, lean only	3 oz.	200	11.0	77	49.5
Cooked, lean & fat	3 oz.	307	25.2	84	73.9
Shoulder					
Cooked, lean only	3 oz.	173	9.2	74	47.9
Cooked, lean & fat,	3 oz.	290	23.0	78	71.1
Liver, braised	3 oz.	187	7.5	426	36.1
Leg, lean, roasted	3 oz.	160	6.0	79	34.0
Pork					
Boston butt, roasted, lean only	3 oz.	233	15.1	81	58.3
Chitterlings, pork, simmered	3 oz.	258	24.4	122	85.1
Chop, lean					
Loin, braised	3 oz.	230	12.0	56	47.0
Rib, lean, braised	3 oz.	230	12.0	0	47.0
Loin, blade, lean only	3 oz.	237	16.3	6	61.9
Pig's feet, pickled	1 oz.	56	4.1	30	66.0
Spareribs, roasted, lean/fat	6 ribs	396	35.0	121	68.4
Tenderloin, roasted, lean	3 oz.	139	4.1	67	25.8

■ Contains less than 20% fat

Item	PORTION	CAL-ORIES	FAT GRAMS	CHOLES-TEROL	% OF FAT
Veal					
Breast, roasted w/bone	3 oz.	256	18.6	100	65.0
Cubed, for stew, braised, lean only	3 oz.	160	3.7	123	20.8
■Cutlet, breaded	3 oz.	115	2.3	14	18.0
Leg, braised					
Lean only	3 oz.	173	4.3	115	22.4
Lean & fat	3 oz.	179	5.4	114	27.1
Loin, braised					
Lean only	3 oz.	192	7.8	106	36.6
Lean & fat	3 oz.	242	14.6	100	54.3
Rib, braised					
Lean only	3 oz.	185	6.6	122	32.1
Lean & fat	3 oz.	213	10.7	118	45.2
Shoulder					
Lean only	3 oz.	145	5.6	97	34.7
Lean & fat	3 oz.	156	7.2	96	41.5
Sirloin, braised					
Lean only	3 oz.	173	5.5	96	28.6
Lean & fat	3 oz.	214	11.2	92	47.1
Organ Meats					
Brains, simmered	3 oz.	136	10.6	1,747	70.1
Heart, simmered	3 oz.	149	4.8	164	28.9
Kidney, simmered	3 oz.	122	2.9	329	21.4
Liver, fried	3 oz.	185	6.8	410	33.1
Pancreas, braised	3 oz.	230	15.0	200	59.0
Thymus, braised	3 oz.	271	21.2	250	70.4
Tongue, simmered	3 oz.	241	17.6	91	65.7
Tripe, cooked	3 oz.	100	5.0	81	45.0
Prepared or Processed Meats					
Bacon, regular, broiled	1 slice	35	3.1	35	79.6

■ Contains less than 20% fat   121

Item	PORTION	CAL-ORIES	FAT GRAMS	CHOLES-TEROL	% OF FAT
Canadian, broiled or fried, drained	1 slice	43	1.8	12	41.3
Cured, broiled or fried, drained	1 slice (.3 oz.)	43	3.7	6	77.4
Bacon, imitation					
Bits	3 oz.	264	25.1	0	85.6
Beef, Sizzlean	2 strips	70	5.0	–	64.3
Breakfast strips, Sizzlean	1 slice	49	3.9	–	71.6
Meatless	1 strip	25	2.4	0	86.4
Pork, Sizzlean	2 strips	90	8.0	–	80.0
Beef jerky	2 oz.	94	2.2	–	21.1
Beef, corned					
Buddig, lean	1 slice	40	2.0	20	45.0
Canned	1 oz.	71	4.2	24	53.2
Cooked	1 oz.	71	5.4	28	68.5
Jellied loaf	2 oz.	87	3.5	27	36.2
Beef, sliced, Buddig, lean	1 slice	40	2.0	–	45.0
Bockwurst, raw, pork/veal	2 oz.	174	15.6	–	80.7
Bologna					
Beef					
Hebrew National	1 oz.	90	8.0	17	80.0
Oscar Mayer	1 oz.	90	8.3	20	83.0
Beef & pork	2 oz.	179	16.0	31	80.4
Chicken, Health Valley	1 slice	85	8.0	13	84.8
Meat					
Lebanon, Seltzer	1 slice	40	2.0	15	45.0
Plain, Oscar Mayer	1 oz.	90	8.3	19	83.0
With cheese, Oscar Mayer	1 slice (.8 oz.)	74	6.8	15	82.7
15% chicken, Smok-A-Roma	1 oz.	90	8.0	–	80.0
■ Turkey, Louis Rich	1 slice	58	4.7	19	17.9

■ Contains less than 20% fat   122

Item	PORTION	CALORIES	FAT GRAMS	CHOLESTEROL	% OF FAT
Bratwurst, cooked, pork	2 oz.	171	14.6	34	76.8
Braunschweiger, pork	2 oz.	204	18.1	88	79.8
Chicken breast					
■ Healthy Choice, smoked	2 oz.	60	1.2	30	18.0
■ Hillshire Farms, oven roasted	2 oz.	50	0.3	20	8.0
Louis Rich, deluxe roasted	2 oz.	60	1.6	28	24.0
Tyson Frozen					
BBQ	3 oz.	100	3.0	35	27.0
Lemon pepper	2.75 oz.	110	3.0	35	24.5
Oriental strips	2.75 oz.	110	3.0	40	24.5
Chicken roll, light meat	2 oz.	90	4.2	28	42.0
Chicken, sliced, Buddig	1 slice	60	4.0	–	60.0
Chorizo, pork & beef	2 oz.	20.0	21.7	–	97.0
Corn dog, frozen, Little Juan	2¾ oz.	231	11.6	–	48.2
Frankfurter					
Bacon & cheddar, Oscar Mayer	1.6 oz.	139	12.3	30	79.6
Beef					
Ball Park	2 oz.	167	16.0	–	86.2
Boar's Head	1 oz.	80	7.0	15	78.7
■ Healthy Choice	1.6 oz.	50	1.0	–	18.0
Hebrew National	1.7 oz.	149	14.0	30	75.2
Oscar Mayer	1.6 oz	143	13.2	30	83.1
Oscar Mayer, light	2 oz.	135	11.0	20	73.3
Beef, lite, Hebrew National	1.7 oz.	120	10.0	–	75.0
Chicken					
Health Valley, weiner	1	96	8.0	49	75.0

Item	PORTION	CAL-ORIES	FAT GRAMS	CHOLES-TEROL	% OF FAT
Perdue	2 oz.	140	11.0	–	70.7
Weaver	2 oz.	115	10.0	–	78.3
Chicken & Cheese, Weaver	2 oz.	145	11.0	–	68.3
With cheese	1.6 oz.	144	13.1	30	81.9
■ Hormel, 97% Fat free	1	45	1.0	10	20.0
Jumbo Frank, Healthy Choice	1	60	2.0	20	30.0
Meat					
Safeway	2 oz.	170	16.0	–	84.7
Smok-A-Roma	2 oz.	140	12.0	–	77.1
Turkey, Empire Kosher	2 oz.	107	9.0	65	75.7
Turkey & Cheese					
Louis Rich	2 oz.	110	9.0	–	73.6
Mr. Turkey	2 oz.	109	9.0	–	74.3
Ham Loaf, glazed	3 oz.	236	14.3	90	54.5
Ham, chopped, canned	3 oz.	203	16.0	42	70.9
Ham, sliced, Buddig, lean	1 slice	50	3.0	–	54.0
Ham, turkey, Buddig	2 oz.	80	4.0	32	36.0
Ham, turkey, Healthy Choice	2 oz.	60	1.6	40	24.0
Ham, turkey, Louis Rich	1 slice	34	0.9	19	31.8
Headcheese	2 oz.	120	9.0	46	67.5
Hot Dog					
Beef	1	176	16.0	34	81.8
Chicken	1	113	8.6	44	68.5
Turkey	1	99	7.8	47	70.9
Healthy Favorites Hot Dog, Oscar Mayer	1	55	1.6	22	26.0
Kielbasa					
Pork & beef	3 oz.	264	23.1	57	78.7

Item	PORTION	CAL-ORIES	FAT GRAMS	CHOLES-TEROL	% OF FAT
Kielbasa, Turkey, Butterball	2 oz.	100	6.0	40	54.0
Hillshire Farm, Polska Flavorseal	1 oz.	95	8.5	–	81.0
Knockwurst, Hebrew National	3 oz.	262	25.0	53	85.9
Liver cheese, pork	3 oz.	259	21.7	148	75.4
Liverwurst, fresh	2 oz.	185	16.2	90	78.8
Mortadella, beef & pork	2 oz.	176	14.4	32	73.6
Pastrami					
Beef	2 oz.	198	16.5	53	75.0
Turkey	2 oz.	69	2.9	31	37.8
Sliced, Buddig, lean	1 slice	40	2.0	–	45.0
Pâté					
Chicken liver, canned	3 oz.	171	11.1	–	58.4
Goose liver, smoked, canned	2 oz.	262	24.9	85	85.5
Pepperoni, pork & beef	1 slice	27	2.4	4	80.0
Pig's feet, pickled	3 oz.	173	13.7	78	71.3
Pork, cooked	3 oz.	256	21.9	51	76.9
Pork, salt, raw	3 oz.	636	68.5	73	96.9
Pork & beef, w/non-fat dry milk	3 oz.	275	23.6	54	77.2
Potted meat, Libby's	3 oz.	181	14.8	–	73.6
Salami					
Beef, Hebrew National	1 oz.	80	7.0	16	78.7
Pork, hard, Oscar Mayer	1 oz.	110	9.3	27	76.1
Turkey, Smok-A-Roma	1 oz.	45	3.0	–	60.0
Turkey, cotto, Louis Rich	1 slice	52	3.7	22	64.0

■ Contains less than 20% fat

Item	PORTION	CAL-ORIES	FAT GRAMS	CHOLES-TEROL	% OF FAT
Sausage					
Brown 'N' Serve, Jones	1 link	100	10.0	–	90.0
German, Smok-A-Roma	4-oz. link	350	32.0	–	82.3
Italian, pork, cooked	1 link	213	17.0	51	71.8
Light, w/rice, Jones	1 link	70	5.5	–	70.0
Polish, pork	2 oz.	185	16.3	40	79.3
Pork, fresh, cooked					
Link	1 link	44	3.7	10	75.7
Patty	1 patty	100	8.4	22	75.6
Smoked or Polish, Eckrich	1	70	6.0	–	77.1
Smoked, beef	2 oz.	177	15.3	38	77.8
Turkey					
Louis Rich	1 oz.	45	3.0	–	60.0
Ohse, breakfast	1 oz.	65	5.3	–	73.4
Vienna, beef & pork, canned	1 link	45	4.0	8	80.0
Scrapple	2 oz.	122	7.7	25	56.8
Spam					
w/cheese chunks, Hormel	2 oz.	174	14.9	–	77.1
Deviled, Hormel	2 oz.	156	13.4	–	77.3
■Turkey breast, smoked, 97% fat free, Healthy Favorites	2 slices	40	0.4	18	9.0
Turkey, sliced, Buddig	2 oz.	100	6.0	30	54.0
■Turkey loaf, breast meat	2 oz.	62	0.9	23	13.1
Turkey roll					
Light meat only	2 oz.	83	4.1	24	44.5
Light & dark meat	2 oz.	84	4.0	31	42.8

■ Contains less than 20% fat   126

Item	PORTION	CAL-ORIES	FAT GRAMS	CHOLES-TEROL	% OF FAT
Turkey spread, Underwood	2 oz.	75	2.0	25	24.0
Weiner					
Oscar Meyer	1	181	16.7	29	83.0
Oscar Meyer, light	2 oz.	131	10.8	30	74.2
Yves, tofu	2 oz.	115	5.0	–	39.1
Miscellaneous					
■Frog legs	4 large	73	0.3	57	7.0
■Snails, raw	1	5	0.1	3	18.0

NUTS, SEEDS & PEANUT BUTTER

Item	PORTION	CAL-ORIES	FAT GRAMS	CHOLES-TEROL	% OF FAT
Almonds					
Raw, natural, Blue Diamond	1 oz.	165	14.9	0	81.3
Roasted, Fisher					
Dry, smoked	1 oz.	160	14.0	0	78.7
Honey roasted	1 oz.	150	14.0	0	84.0
Beechnuts, shelled	1 oz.	163	14.2	0	78.4
Brazil nuts, medium	4	115	11.6	0	90.8
Cashews, roasted					
Dry, Fisher	1 oz.	160	13.0	0	73.1
Honey, Planters	1 oz.	170	12.0	0	63.5
Oil, Planters	1 oz.	170	14.0	0	74.1
■Chestnuts, fresh	2 tb.	39	0.4	0	9.2
Coconut					
Raw, not packed	2 tb.	35	3.4	0	87.4
Dried, sweetened, shredded	1 tb.	29	2.1	0	65.2
Hazelnuts, shelled, whole	2 tb.	107	10.6	0	89.2
Macadamia, dried	2 tb.	118	12.4	0	94.6
Mixed, roasted					
Dry, Fisher	1 oz.	170	15.0	0	79.4
Honey, w/peanuts, Fisher	1 oz.	150	13.0	0	78.0

■ Contains less than 20% fat   127

Item	PORTION	CAL-ORIES	FAT GRAMS	CHOLES-TEROL	% OF FAT
Oil, Planters	1 oz.	180	16.0	0	80.0
Peanuts, raw, w/o shell	2 tb.	114	9.9	0	78.2
Peanuts, roasted					
In shell	1 cup	209	17.7	0	77.0
With oil	½ cup	450	35.0	0	70.0
Dry roasted, Planters	1 oz.	160	13.9	–	78.2
Honey roasted, Planters	1 oz.	170	13.0	0	68.8
Peanuts, cocktail, Planters	1 oz.	170	14.0	0	74.1
Peanut butter					
Crunchy, Peter Pan	1 tb.	90	8.0	0	80.0
Extra crunchy, Jif	1 tb.	93	7.8	0	75.5
Smooth					
Estee, low sodium	1 tb.	100	8.0	0	72.0
Peter Pan	1 tb.	90	8.0	0	80.0
Peanut butter & jelly, Bama	1 tb.	75	3.5	–	42.0
Peanuts, Spanish, oil roasted, Fisher	1 oz.	170	14.0	0	74.1
Pecans					
Raw, Fisher	1 oz.	200	20.0	0	90.0
Roasted					
Dry, Fisher	1 oz.	170	18.0	0	95.3
Honey, Eagle	1 oz.	200	19.0	0	85.5
Pine, pignolia	2 tb.	103	10.1	0	88.3
Pistachios, Dole					
Natural, shelled	1 oz.	90	7.0	0	70.0
Roasted, shelled	1 oz.	163	14.0	0	77.3
Poppy seeds	2 tb.	94	7.8	0	74.7
Pumpkin seed kernels, dry	2 tb.	93	7.9	0	76.5
Sesame seeds, dry, whole	2 tb.	103	8.9	0	77.8

■ Contains less than 20% fat

Item	PORTION	CAL-ORIES	FAT GRAMS	CHOLES-TEROL	% OF FAT
Sunflower seeds	2 tb.	103	8.9	0	77.8
Trail mix					
w/coconut	2 tb.	143	11.0	0	69.2
w/seeds, nuts, and carob	2 tb.	88	5.1	0	51.0
Walnuts					
Black	2 tb.	95	8.8	0	83.4
Persian or English, shelled, halves	2 tb.	80	7.7	0	86.6

PASTA & NOODLES

Item	PORTION	CAL-ORIES	FAT GRAMS	CHOLES-TEROL	% OF FAT
■Macaroni, regular					
Cooked	1 cup	197	0.9	0	4.1
Cooked, al dente	1 cup	155	0.6	0	3.5
Ronzoni, dry	2 oz.	210	1.0	–	4.3
Spirals, cooked	1 cup	189	0.9	0	4.3
■Macaroni, whole wheat, cooked	1 cup	174	0.8	0	4.1
Noodles, chow mein, canned	1 cup	237	13.8	0	52.4
■Noodles, egg					
Cooked	1 cup	213	2.4	53	10.1
Dry	2 oz.	216	2.4	54	10.0
■Noodles, egg, no yolk, Penna. Dutch	2 oz.	210	1.0	0	4.3
■Noodles, no egg, fettucini, cooked	1 cup	197	0.9	0	4.1
■Noodles, lasagna, cooked	1 cup	197	0.9	0	4.1
■Noodles, rice, cooked,	1 cup	277	2.6	0	8.4
Noodle Roni					
With herb butter, Quaker	1 cup	240	13.0	–	48.7
Parmesano, Quaker	1 cup	250	14.0	–	50.4

■ Contains less than 20% fat

Item	PORTION	CALORIES	FAT GRAMS	CHOLESTEROL	% OF FAT
■Pasta, fresh, w/egg, refrigerated, cooked	3 oz.	297	2.4	75	7.3
■Pasta, fresh, angel hair, DiGiorno	3 oz.	250	3.0	0	11.0
Pasta Sauces, see Sauces & Gravies p. 141					
■Spaghetti					
Cooked	1 cup	197	0.9	0	4.1
Cooked al dente	1 cup	155	0.6	0	3.5
Amaranth, dry, Health Valley	2 oz.	170	1.0	0	5.5
Oat Bran, dry, Health Valley	2 oz.	120	1.0	0	7.5
Ronzoni, dry	2 oz.	210	1.0	–	4.3
Vegetable tri-color, dry, Creamettes	2 oz.	210	1.0	–	4.3
Whole wheat, dry, Health Valley	2 oz.	170	1.0	0	5.5
Whole wheat, spinach, dry, Hodgeson Mills	2 oz.	200	1.0	–	4.5
Spaghetti twist, w/sauce, Buitoni	15-oz. can	300	8.0	0	24.0

POULTRY

Chicken
Breast, baked or broiled

■ No skin	½ breast	142	3.0	73	19.0
With skin	½ breast	193	7.6	82	35.4
Breast, fried					
No skin, boneless	½ breast	161	4.1	78	23.0
With skin	½ breast	338	17.0	111	45.3
Canned, white meat, Swanson	2.5 oz.	100	4.0	–	36.0
Capon, w/skin, roasted	3 oz.	195	9.9	73	45.7

■ Contains less than 20% fat   130

Item	PORTION	CAL-ORIES	FAT GRAMS	CHOLES-TEROL	% OF FAT
Fryer, dark meat, no skin					
Fried	3 oz.	203	9.9	82	44.0
Roasted	3 oz.	174	8.3	79	42.9
Stewed	3 oz.	163	7.6	75	42.0
Fryer, dark meat, w/skin					
Floured, fried	3 oz.	242	14.2	78	52.8
Roasted	3 oz.	215	13.4	77	56.1
Stewed	3 oz.	198	12.5	70	56.8
Fryer, white meat, no skin					
Roasted	3 oz.	147	3.8	72	23.3
Stewed	3 oz.	135	3.4	65	22.7
Fryer, white meat, w/skin					
Fried	3 oz.	236	13.1	71	50.0
Roasted	3 oz.	189	9.2	71	44.8
Stewed	3 oz.	171	8.5	63	44.7
Fryer, heart, sim-mered	3 oz.	157	6.7	206	38.4
Fryer, thigh, w/skin, floured, fried	3 oz.	223	12.7	82	51.2
Fryer, wing meat, w/skin					
Fried	3 oz.	276	18.5	67	60.3
Roasted	3 oz.	247	16.5	71	60.1
Stewed	3 oz.	100	6.7	28	60.3
Giblets, cooked	3 oz.	134	4.0	334	26.9
Gizzards, simmered,	3 oz.	130	3.1	165	21.5
Leg, baked or broiled					
No skin, drumstick	1	76	2.5	41	30.0
With skin, drum-stick	1	112	5.8	105	46.0
Leg, fried, w/skin	1	120	8.7	99	65.0
Liver, cooked	3 oz.	134	4.6	537	31.0
Roaster, meat only, roasted	3 oz.	142	5.6	64	35.5
Stewing, meat only, stewed					
No skin	3 oz.	202	10.1	71	45.0
With skin	3 oz.	242	16.0	67	59.5

■ Contains less than 20% fat   131

Item	PORTION	CAL- ORIES	FAT GRAMS	CHOLES- TEROL	% OF FAT
Thigh, cooked					
No skin	1	105	5.4	48	46.3
With skin	1	153	9.6	58	56.5
Game					
Cornish game hen	3 oz.	206	12.0	60	52.4
Duck					
Domesticated, roasted	3 oz.	171	9.4	76	49.5
Wild, raw	3 oz.	105	3.6	–	30.8
Goose, domesticated					
Liver, raw	1	124	4.0	550	29.0
Roasted					
No skin	3 oz.	202	10.8	82	48.1
With skin	3 oz.	259	18.6	77	64.6
Guinea hen, raw	3 oz.	94	2.1	54	20.1
Pheasant, raw	3 oz.	113	3.1	–	24.7
Quail, raw	3 oz.	114	3.9	–	30.8
Squab, raw	3 oz.	121	6.4	–	47.6
Turkey					
Light and dark, roasted, meat only					
No skin	3 oz.	145	4.2	65	26.1
With skin	3 oz.	177	8.3	70	42.2
Breast, meat only, raw	3 oz.	94	0.5	53	4.8
Breast, w/skin	3 oz.	161	6.3	63	35.2
Breast, commercial					
BBQ, cooked, Louis Rich	3 oz.	114	3.7	30	29.2
Honey cured ham, Louis Rich	3 oz.	75	2.1	42	25.0
Oven-roasted, Louis Rich	3 oz.	92	2.7	32	26.4
Smoked, Louis Rich	3 oz.	94	2.1	37	20.1

■ Contains less than 20% fat

Item	PORTION	CAL-ORIES	FAT GRAMS	CHOLES-TEROL	% OF FAT
Dark meat, cooked					
No skin	3 oz.	159	6.1	72	34.5
With skin	3 oz.	188	9.8	76	47.0
Leg, cooked, w/skin	3 oz.	177	8.3	72	42.2
White meat, cooked					
■ No skin	3 oz.	134	2.7	59	18.1
With skin	3 oz.	168	7.1	65	38.0
Canned, Swanson	2.5 oz.	80	1.0	–	11.5
Wing, w/skin, cooked	3 oz.	195	10.6	69	49.0
Ground					
Cooked	3 oz.	195	11.7	59	54.0
Fresh, Louis Rich	3 oz.	156	6.3	75	36.1
Fresh, breast, The Turkey Store	3.5 oz.	100	1.0	56	9.0
Ham, turkey, cured, thigh	3 oz.	109	4.3	0	35.5
Liver, simmered	1	131	4.6	484	31.6
Sausage, breakfast, cooked, Louis Rich	3 oz.	180	11.7	71	58.5
Sliced					
Carl Buddig	3 oz.	150	9.0	45	50.0
■ White meat, raw, The Turkey Store	3.5 oz.	100	1.0	60	9.0
■Spread, Underwood	2 oz.	75	1.0	25	10.5
Wing, drumettes, cooked, Louis Rich	3 oz.	160	6.8	62	38.3

RICE & GRAINS

Rice					
■Brown, cooked	½ cup	108	0.9	0	0.8
Cakes					
■ Chico San	1	36	0.2	0	5.0

■ Contains less than 20% fat

Item	PORTION	CALORIES	FAT GRAMS	CHOLESTEROL	% OF FAT
Hain, mini					
■ Plain	1	50	0.2	–	3.6
Barbecue	1	70	3.0	0	38.6
■ Heart Lovers	1	35	0.0	0	0.0
■ Pritikin	1	35	0.0	0	0.0
■Fried, canned, La Choy	½ cup	135	1.0	0	19.0
Mix					
■ Au gratin, herb, Success	½ cup	100	0.0	–	0.0
■ Beef, Lipton, & sauce	¼ pkg.	120	0.5	0	3.7
■ Broccoli and cheese, Success	½ cup	120	1.0	–	9.6
■ Brown and wild, Success	½ cup	100	0.0	–	0.0
Chicken					
■ Lipton, & sauce	¼ pkg.	125	1.1	0	7.9
■ Rice-A-Roni, prepared	½ cup	107	0.7	–	5.8
Milanese, risotto, Knorr, prepared	½ cup	130	3.0	–	20.8
■Curry rice, Near East	½ cup	60	0.2	0	3.0
■Long grain & wild rice, Near East	½ cup	60	0.2	0	3.0
Pilaf					
With margarine	½ cup	134	3.2	–	21.5
■ Brown rice, Near East	½ cup	60	0.4	–	6.0
■ Mix, dry, Near East	1 oz.	102	0.0	–	0.0
Wheat mix, Near East	½ cup	170	6.0	–	31.8
■Risotto, Ferrara, dry	2 oz.	200	4.0	0	18.0
Spanish					
Homemade	½ cup	97	3.3	0	30.6
■ Birds Eye	½ cup	123	0.5	0	3.7
Lipton	½ cup	140	3.0	–	19.3

■ Contains less than 20% fat   134

Item	PORTION	CAL-ORIES	FAT GRAMS	CHOLES-TEROL	% OF FAT
■ Near East	½ cup	60	0.2	0	3.0
■ Rice-A-Roni	½ cup	80	0.7	–	7.9
■ Van Kamp's, canned	½ cup	75	1.5	–	18.0
■White, cooked	½ cup	132	0.3	0	2.0
■White, long grain					
Instant cooked	½ cup	81	0.1	0	1.1
Minute Rice	⅔ cup	120	0.0	0	0.0
■Wild					
Uncooked	½ cup	286	0.9	0	2.8
Cooked	½ cup	83	0.3	0	3.2

Other Grains

Item	PORTION	CAL-ORIES	FAT GRAMS	CHOLES-TEROL	% OF FAT
■Amaranth, cooked	½ cup	62	1.0	0	15.0
■Barley, pearled, cooked	½ cup	97	0.3	0	2.8
■Bulgar, dry	1 oz.	97	0.4	0	3.7
■Couscous, medium grain	1 cup	196	0.0	0	0.0
■Kamut	½ cup	59	0.4	0	7.0
■Kashi pilaf	½ cup	177	1.0	0	5.5
■Quinoa, cooked	½ cup	62	1.0	0	15.0
■Tabouleh, wheat salad mix, Near East	½ cup	94	0.2	0	3.0
■Wheat pilaf, Near East	½ cup	60	0.2	0	3.0

SALADS

Item	PORTION	CAL-ORIES	FAT GRAMS	CHOLES-TEROL	% OF FAT
Bacon bits, imitation	2 tb.	56	5.3	0	85.2
■Beans, garbanzo, dried, cooked, and drained	2 tb.	34	0.5	0	13.2
■Broccoli, raw, chopped	2 tb.	3	0.0	0	0.0

■ Contains less than 20% fat

135

Item	PORTION	CAL-ORIES	FAT GRAMS	CHOLES-TEROL	% OF FAT
Caesar, w/oil & egg dressing	2 cup	210	21.0	2	90.0
■Carrots, raw, diced	2 tb.	7	0.0	0	0.0
Carrot & raisin, made w/mayonnaise	½ cup	164	11.3	15	62.0
Cheese, cheddar, shredded	2 tb.	57	4.7	15	74.2
Cheese, cottage	2 tb.	27	1.2	4	40.0
Chef's, w/ham & turkey, no dressing	3 oz.	390	21.9	234	50.5
Chicken, w/mayonnaise	½ cup	221	15.9	122	64.7
Coleslaw					
Regular, made w/mayonnaise	½ cup	41	1.6	5	35.1
■ Diet, no salt, vinegar dressing	½ cup	32	0.2	0	5.6
Croutons	½ oz.	30	1.0	0	30.0
■Cucumbers, raw, not pared	2 tb.	2	0.0	0	0.0
Egg, hard-cooked, chopped	2 tb.	26	1.8	72	62.3
■Lettuce	1 cup	7	0.1	0	12.8
Lobster, w/mayonnaise	½ cup	314	26.3	295	75.4
Macaroni, made w/mayonnaise	½ cup	349	23.4	136	60.3
■Mushrooms, raw	2 tb.	2	0.0	0	0.0
■Onions, raw, chopped	2 tb.	8	0.0	0	0.0
Pasta prima vera	1 cup	149	5.9	–	35.0
*■Pasta w/seafood	1 cup	243	1.8	70	7.0
■Peppers, green, raw, strips	½ cup	3	0.0	0	0.0
Potato, w/mayonnaise & hard-cooked egg	½ cup	237	17.3	47	65.0

Item	PORTION	CALORIES	FAT GRAMS	CHOLESTEROL	% OF FAT
Potato, German, General Mills	½ cup	134	3.7	–	24.8
Sunflower seeds	2 tb.	103	8.9	0	77.8
Tabouleh salad w/oil	½ cup	173	9.5	0	49.0
Three bean					
w/oil dressing	½ cup	112	5.8	0	46.6
■ w/o oil	½ cup	90	0.3	0	3.0
Tomatoes, fresh, chopped	2 tb.	5	0.0	0	0.0
■Tuna, made w/mayonnaise	½ cup	273	20.3	117	66.9
Turkey, made w/mayonnaise	½ cup	211	14.6	114	62.3
Waldorf, made w/mayonnaise & nuts	½ cup	165	13.6	9	74.2
■Wheat salad, Tabouleh, prepared, Near East	½ cup	73	0.0	–	0.0

SALAD DRESSINGS

Item	PORTION	CALORIES	FAT GRAMS	CHOLESTEROL	% OF FAT
Bacon & tomato, Henri's	1 tb.	70	6.0	–	77.1
Blue cheese					
Henri's	1 tb.	60	5.0	–	75.0
Kraft, Wish-Bone, chunky	1 tb.	76	7.6	4	90.0
Walden Farms	1 tb.	27	2.0	5	66.7
Blue cheese, low calorie					
■ Estee	1 tb.	8	0.0	0	0.0
Henri's	1 tb.	35	2.0	–	51.4
■ Hidden Valley Take Heart	1 tb.	12	0.0	0	0.0
Kraft Roka	1 tb.	16	1.0	5	56.2
Kraft	1 tb.	59	5.8	11	88.5
Wish-Bone	1 tb.	40	3.7	0	83.2

■ Contains less than 20% fat

Item	PORTION	CALORIES	FAT GRAMS	CHOLESTEROL	% OF FAT
■Blue cheese mix, dietetic, Good Seasons	1 tb.	3	0.0	0	0.0
Blue cheese & herbs, mix, Good Seasons	1 tb.	58	6.0	6	93.1
Buttermilk, Hain	1 tb.	70	7.0	0	90.0
Buttermilk mix, Good Seasons, farm style	1 tb.	58	6.0	6	93.1
■Buttermilk mix, no oil, Hain	1 tb.	11	0.0	0	0.0
Caesar, Wish-Bone	1 tb.	78	8.1	1	93.5
■Caesar, low-calorie, low-fat, Weight Watchers	¾-oz. pkt.	6	0.0	–	0.0
Caesar, low-sodium, Hain	1 tb.	60	6.0	0	90.0
■Caesar mix, no oil, Hain	1 tb.	6	0.0	0	0.0
Coleslaw, commercial	1 tb.	57	4.9	4	77.4
Cucumber, Wish-Bone	1 tb.	80	8.0	0	90.0
■Cucumber, low-calorie, non-fat, Herb Magic	1 tb.	8	0.0	0	0.0
■Dijon, creamy, low-calorie, Estee	1 tb.	8	0.0	5	0.0
Dijon vinaigrette, Wish-Bone	1 tb.	60	6.1	0	91.5
French					
Homemade	1 tb.	87	9.6	–	99.3
Henri's, hearty	1 tb.	70	6.0	–	77.1
Kraft, Catalina	1 tb.	65	5.6	0	77.5
Kraft, regular	1 tb.	59	5.7	0	86.9
Seven Seas, creamy,	1 tb.	61	6.0	0	88.5

■ Contains less than 20% fat

138

Item	PORTION	CAL-ORIES	FAT GRAMS	CHOLES-TEROL	% OF FAT
■French, low-fat					
Estee	1 tb.	4	0.0	0	0.0
Kraft Catalina, re-duced calorie	1 tb.	16	.6	0	33.7
Kraft Free	1 tb.	20	0.0	0	0.0
■ Medford Farms Chef's Lite	1 tb.	7	0.0	0	0.0
Pritikin	1 tb.	10	0.0	0	0.0
Walden Farms, re-duced calorie	1 tb.	33	2.0	2	54.5
■ Weight Watchers	1 tb.	10	0.0	0	0.0
Western Lite	1 tb.	35	1.0	0	25.7
Wish-Bone, red	1 tb.	30	0.4	0	12.0
■French mix, no oil, Hain	1 tb.	12	0.0	0	0.0
Garlic, Wish-Bone, creamy	1 tb.	74	8.0	0	97.3
■Garlic, low-fat, Estee	1 tb.	2	0.0	0	0.0
Garlic & cheese, mix, Good Seasons	1 tb.	72	7.5	0	94.4
■Garlic & cheese, mix, no oil, Hain	1 tb.	6	0.0	0	0.0
Green Goddess, Kraft	1 tb.	70	7.4	09	95.1
Italian					
Bernstein's	1 tb.	32	1.0	0	28.1
Kraft, creamy	1 tb.	55	5.5	1	90.0
Kraft	1 tb.	73	7.7	0	94.9
■ Walden Farms	1 tb.	9	0.0	0	0.0
Italian, low-calorie					
■ Good Seasons, zesty, light,	1 tb.	25	3.0	0	100.0
■ Kraft	1 tb.	7	0.0	0	0.0
Wish-Bone	1 tb.	1	0.0	0	0.0
■Italian, low-fat					
Hidden Valley Take Heart	1 tb.	16	0.0	0	0.0
Kraft Free	1 tb.	6	0.0	0	0.0

■ Contains less than 20% fat   139

Item	PORTION	CAL- ORIES	FAT GRAMS	CHOLES- TEROL	% OF FAT
No oil	1 tb.	8	0.0	0	0.0
Oil free, Kraft	1 tb.	4	0.0	0	0.0
Pritikin	1 tb.	4	0.0	–	0.0
Walden Farms, w/cheese	1 tb.	15	0.0	3	0.0
Wish-Bone, creamy, light,	1 tb.	6	0.0	0	0.0
■Italian, mix					
Good Seasons	1 each	3	0.0	0	0.0
■Italian, mix, low-fat					
Good Seasons	1 each	3	0.0	0	0.0
No oil, Good Seasons, prepared	1 tb.	7	0.0	0	0.0
Wish-bone, fat free, Healthy Sensation	1 tb.	6	0.0	0	0.0
Italian, w/sour cream, Kraft	1 tb.	55	5.5	1	90.0
Mayonnaise					
Regular	1 tb.	99	10.9	8	99.1
Hellman's	1 tb.	98	10.8	10	99.2
Mayonnaise, imitation	1 tb.	35	2.9	4	74.6
Mayonnaise, low-calorie					
Kraft	1 tb.	44	4.6	6	94.1
Light 'N' Lively	1 tb.	40	4.0	5	90.0
■Mayonnaise, Kraft Free	1 tb.	12	0.0	0	0.0
Miracle Whip	1 tb.	69	6.9	5	90.0
Olive oil, light, Wish-Bone	1 tb.	16	1.0	0	56.2
Ranch					
Regular	1 tb.	58	5.7	5	88.4
Newman's Own	1 tb.	90	9.0	5	90.0
Ranch, low-calorie, Take Heart, Hidden Valley	1 tb.	20	1.0	0	45.0

■ Contains less than 20% fat

Item	PORTION	CAL-ORIES	FAT GRAMS	CHOLES-TEROL	% OF FAT
■Ranch, low-fat					
Kraft Free	1 tb.	16	0.0	0	0.0
Pritikin	1 tb.	18	0.0	0	0.0
Roka, reduced-calorie, Kraft	1 tb.	14	0.9	3	57.9
Russian	1 tb.	76	7.8	–	92.4
Russian, low-fat	1 tb.	23	0.7	1	27.4
Sesame seed	1 tb.	62	5.8	0	84.2
Sweet & sour, Sysco Classic	1 tb.	59	5.9	0	90.0
Thousand Island, Kraft	1 tb.	56	5.1	7	81.9
Thousand Island, low-calorie					
■ Kraft Free	1 tb.	6	0.0	0	0.0
■ Slim Fast	1 tb.	18	0.1	0	2.5
Take Heart, Hidden Valley	1 tb.	29	2.1	6	65.2
Wish-Bone	1 tb.	35	3.0	10	77.1
Thousand Island, low-fat,					
■ Kraft Free	1 tb.	20	0.0	0	0.0
Vinegar and oil, homemade	1 tb.	70	7.8	0	100.0
Vinaigrette					
■ Seven Seas Free, red wine	1 tb.	6	0.0	0	0.0
■ Newman's Own, olive oil	1 tb.	80	9.0	0	100.0

SAUCES & GRAVIES

Sauces
BBQ

Item	PORTION	CAL-ORIES	FAT GRAMS	CHOLES-TEROL	% OF FAT
■ Estee, low sodium	2 tb.	36	0.0	0	0.0
Hunt's, original or hickory	2 tb.	40	1.0	0	22.5
■ La Choy, oriental	2 tb.	32	0.5	0	14.1
■ Open Pit, original	2 tb.	45	0.4	–	8.0

■ Contains less than 20% fat   141

Item	PORTION	CAL-ORIES	FAT GRAMS	CHOLES-TEROL	% OF FAT
Bearnaise, mix, Knorr	2 tb.	85	8.5	–	90.0
Cheese, Snow's, Welsh Rarebit	½ cup	170	11.0	–	58.2
Chili					
La Victoria, green	2 tb.	6	0.5	–	75.0
■ Ortega, hot	2 tb.	9	0.1	0	10.0
■Chutney					
Apple	2 tb.	82	0.0	–	0.0
Tomato	2 tb.	62	0.0	–	0.0
Clam, red, Progresso	½ cup	70	3.0	–	38.6
Clam, white					
Contadina, deluxe	2 tb.	57	4.4	–	69.5
Progresso, authen-tic	½ cup	130	9.0	19	62.3
■Cranberry, home-made, sweet-ened	2 tb.	62	0.1	0	1.4
Demi-glace, mix, pre-pared, Knorr	2 fl. oz.	30	1.0	–	30.0
■Enchilada, Rosarita	2 oz.	13	0.0	–	0.0
Grilling & broiling, Knorr					
Chardonnay	1 oz.	31	2.5	–	72.6
Tequila lime	1 oz.	33	1.9	–	52.7
Hollandaise					
Homemade	2 tb.	137	14.4	142	94.6
Frozen, made w/vegetable oil	2 tb.	88	8.5	24	86.9
Knorr					
Microwave	1 oz.	50	5.0	–	90.0
Mix, prepared	2 oz.	170	18.0	–	95.3
■Marinara, Enrico's	4 oz.	60	1.0	–	15.0
■Marinara #2, Pritikin	½ cup	53	0.4	0	6.8
Mushroom, dry, made w/milk	2 tb.	28	1.3	4	41.8
■Orange, mandarin, La Choy	2 tb.	46	0.0	0	0.0

Item	PORTION	CAL-ORIES	FAT GRAMS	CHOLES-TEROL	% OF FAT
Parmesano, Knorr, microwave	1 oz.	31	2.3	–	67.1
Pepper, mix, prepared, Knorr	2 oz.	20	0.6	–	27.0
Pesto, homemade	2 tb.	169	15.8	4	84.1
■Picante, Pace, original	2 tb.	12	0.1	0	7.5
Pizza Quick, Ragu	3 tb.	35	2.0	0	51.4
■Plum, tangy, La Choy	1 oz.	44	0.1	0	2.0
■Salsa brava, La Victoria	2 tb.	12	0.2	–	15.0
■Salsa verde, Old El Paso	2 tb.	10	0.0	0	0.0
■Seafood cocktail	¼ cup	70	0.0	–	0.0
Sour cream, dehydrated, w/milk	1 tb.	32	1.9	6	53.4
■Soy					
Kikkoman	2 tb.	24	0.0	0	0.0
La Choy	2 tb.	2	0.0	0	0.0
Spaghetti, w/lobster, rock, Progresso	½ cup	120	8.0	10	60.0
Spaghetti, w/meat					
■ Enrico's, all varieties	½ cup	60	1.0	0	15.0
Hunt's	½ cup	70	2.0	2	25.7
Newman's Own	½ cup	70	2.0	0	25.0
Prego, meat flavored	½ cup	140	6.0	39	38.6
Ragu, extra thick, zesty	½ cup	111	11.9	–	96.5
Ragu, Old World Style	½ cup	80	4.0	0	45.0
Town House	½ cup	80	3.0	2	33.7
Spaghetti, meatless					
Hunt's, traditional	½ cup	60	2.1	0	30.0
■ Chef Boyardee	½ cup	60	1.0	–	15.0
Prego	½ cup	130	5.0	–	34.6
■ Pritikin	½ cup	60	0.0	0	0.0

■ Contains less than 20% fat   143

Item	PORTION	CAL-ORIES	FAT GRAMS	CHOLES-TEROL	% OF FAT
Progresso	½ cup	110	5.0	2	40.9
Ragu, Chunky Garden	½ cup	80	4.0	0	45.0
Spaghetti, mushroom					
Prego, extra chunky, & tomato	½ cup	110	5.0	–	40.9
■ Pritikin	½ cup	60	0.0	0	0.0
Progresso	½ cup	110	5.0	5	40.9
■ Weight Watchers, mushroom flavored	½ cup	60	0.0	–	0.0
Spaghetti, primavera, creamy, Progresso	½ cup	190	17.0	54	80.5
Spaghetti, w/sausage & green pepper, Prego, extra chunky	½ cup	160	8.0	–	45.0
Spaghetti, Sicilian style, Progresso	½ cup	30	2.5	0	75.0
■Spaghetti, Ragu, Today's Recipe	½ cup	50	1.0	0	18.0
■Spaghetti, tomato & basil, Prego	½ cup	100	2.0	–	18.0
■Steak					
A-1	1 tb.	12	0.0	–	0.0
Estee	1 tb.	14	0.0	–	0.0
Stir-fry, Kikkoman	2 tb.	96	0.0	0	0.0
■Szechuan, hot & spicy, La Choy	1 oz.	48	.2	0	3.7
Tabasco	1 tb.	2	0.1	0	45.0
■Taco, La Victoria, green	2 tb.	8	0.0	0	0.0
Tartar					
Kraft	1 tb.	72	7.6	7	95.0
Weight Watchers	1 tb.	35	3.0	5	68.6

■ Contains less than 20% fat   144

Item	PORTION	CAL-ORIES	FAT GRAMS	CHOLES-TEROL	% OF FAT
■Teriyaki, Kikkoman	2 tb.	30	0.0	0	0.0
■Tomato, canned, Contadina	½ cup	57	0.0	0	0.0
White sauce, medium	2 tb.	54	4.1	5	68.0
■Worcestershire	1 tb.	12	0.0	0	0.0
Gravies					
■Au jus					
Canned, Franco-American	¼ cup	10	0.0	–	0.0
Mix, prepared, Lawry's	¼ cup	21	0.4	–	17.1
Beef, canned, Franco-American	¼ cup	25	1.0	–	36.0
Brown					
Canned					
■ Estee, dietetic	¼ cup	14	0.0	0	0.0
■ La Choy	¼ cup	140	0.0	0	0.0
Dehydrated, w/water	2 tb.	1	0.0	0	0.0
Mix, prepared					
French's	¼ cup	20	1.0	0	45.0
Knorr	¼ cup	25	0.9	0	32.4
Chicken					
Canned					
■ Estee, & herbs, dietetic	¼ cup	20	0.0	0	0.0
Franco-American, giblet	¼ cup	30	2.0	–	60.0
■ Dehydrated, made w/water	2 tb.	10	0.2	0	18.0
Mix, prepared, Pillsbury	¼ cup	25	1.0	–	36.0
Homestyle, mix, prepared					
French's	¼ cup	20	1.0	0	45.0
■ Pillsbury	¼ cup	15	0.0	–	0.0

■ Contains less than 20% fat   145

Item	PORTION	CAL-ORIES	FAT GRAMS	CHOLES-TEROL	% OF FAT
Mushroom					
Canned, Franco-American	¼ cup	25	1.0	–	36.0
■ Dehydrated, made w/water	2 tb.	9	0.1	0	10.0
Pork					
Canned, Franco-American	¼ cup	40	3.0	–	67.5
■ Dehydrated, made w/water	2 tb.	10	0.2	0	18.0
Turkey					
Canned, Franco-American	¼ cup	30	2.0	–	60.0
■ Dehydrated, made w/water	1 tb.	11	0.2	0	16.4
White					
*■ Homemade	2 tb.	38	2.8	2	14.7
Ready-to-serve, General Mills	2 tb.	24	1.3	–	48.7

SNACKS

Item	PORTION	CAL-ORIES	FAT GRAMS	CHOLES-TEROL	% OF FAT
Corn Chips					
Corn Snackers, Weight Watchers	1 oz.	121	4.0	0	29.8
Fritos	1 oz.	150	10.0	0	60.0
Tortilla chips					
Black bean, Garden	1 oz.	130	7.0	0	48.5
■ No oil, Guiltless Gourmet	1 oz.	110	1.4	0	11.5
Doritos	1 oz.	140	6.0	0	38.6
Tostitos	1 oz.	140	8.0	0	51.4
■ Happy Heart, no oil	1 oz.	108	1.0	0	8.3
Health Valley	1 oz.	160	11.0	0	61.9

■ Contains less than 20% fat   146   * See page xxxii

Item	PORTION	CAL-ORIES	FAT GRAMS	CHOLES-TEROL	% OF FAT
Dips					
Avocado, Kraft	2 tb.	50	4.0	0	72.0
Bacon & horseradish, Kraft	2 tb.	60	5.0	–	75.0
■Black bean, Guiltless	1 oz.	25	0.0	0	0.0
Blue cheese, Kraft, premium	2 tb.	45	4.0	10	80.0
■Cheddar Queso, Guiltless	1 oz.	22	0.0	0	0.0
Chili, La Victoria	2 tb.	12	1.0	–	75.0
Chili bean, Old El Paso	2 tb.	16	1.0	–	56.2
Clam, Kraft	2 tb.	60	4.0	10	60.0
Enchilada Dip, Frito's	1 oz.	35	1.2	1	30.8
Guacamole, Calavo	1 oz.	55	4.0	0	65.4
Hot bean, Hain	2 tb.	34	1.0	1	26.5
■Jalapeño, Wise	2 tb.	24	0.0	–	0.0
Onion, French					
■ Hain	2 tb.	34	0.4	1	10.6
Kraft	2 tb.	60	4.0	0	60.0
■Picante, Wise	2 tb.	12	0.0	–	0.0
Spinach Dip, w/sour cream and mayo	2 tb.	74	7.1	10	71.5
Taco, Old El Paso	2 tb.	14	1.0	–	64.3
Popcorn					
Fresh					
■ Air popped	1 cup	23	0.3	0	11.7
Popped w/oil and salt	1 cup	41	2.0	0	43.9
Microwave					
plain	1 cup	67	3.7	0	49.7
buttered	1 cup	67	3.7	–	49.7
Orville Redenbacher's, natural	1 cup	33	2.0	0	54.5

■ Contains less than 20% fat

Item	PORTION	CAL-ORIES	FAT GRAMS	CHOLES-TEROL	% OF FAT
Packaged					
Regular					
Cape Cod	1 cup	48	3.0	0	56.2
Eagle	1 cup	48	3.6	2	67.5
Weight Watchers, low sodium	1 cup	36	1.8	–	45.0
Caramel coated, Old Dutch	1 cup	33	0.2	–	5.4
Cheese coated					
Cape Cod	1 cup	48	3.0	2	56.2
Weight Watchers	1 cup	30	1.8	–	54.0
Potato Chips					
Barbecue					
Delta Gold, mesquite flavored	1 oz.	160	11.0	0	61.9
Eagle, crunchy or Louisiana	1 oz.	150	8.0	0	48.0
Wise Ridgies, cholesterol free	1 oz.	150	10.0	–	60.0
Light, Pringles	1 oz.	148	8.2	0	49.9
Plain					
Cape Cod	1 oz.	150	8.0	0	48.0
Eagle	1 oz.	150	10.0	0	60.0
Hawaiian	1 oz.	150	8.0	0	48.0
Pringles	1 oz.	160	11.0	0	61.9
Regular					
Lay's	1 oz.	150	10.0	0	60.0
Pringles	1 oz.	160	11.0	0	61.9
Ruffles	1 oz.	150	10.0	0	60.9
Sour cream					
Cape Cod, & dill	1 oz.	150	8.0	0	48.0
Eagle, & onion	1 oz.	150	10.0	1	60.0
Ruffles	1 oz.	150	9.0	0	54.0

■ Contains less than 20% fat

Item	PORTION	CALORIES	FAT GRAMS	CHOLESTEROL	% OF FAT
■**Pretzels**					
Regular					
Eagle	1 oz.	110	2.0	0	16.4
Mister Salty					
Dutch	1	55	0.5	–	8.2
Logs	1	12	0.1	–	7.5
Sticks, Veri-Thin	1	2	.02	–	9.0
Twists	1	22	0.4	–	16.4
Unsalted, Estee	1	7	0.0	0	0.0
No fat, thick, Snyder's	1	101	0.0	0	0.0
Soft, commercial	1	145	0.0	0	0.0
■Whole-wheat, mini, Pritikin	19	110	1.5	0	12.0
Other Snacks					
Bagel chips	1 oz.	149	8.8	0	53.0
■Bagel chips, King David's	1 oz.	100	0.0	0	0.0
Bugles	1 oz.	152	8.1	–	50.0
Cheese curls, Ultra Slim Fast	1 oz.	110	3.0	0	25.0
Cheese Straws	1 oz.	128	8.4	–	59.1
Cheetos					
Crunchy	1 oz.	160	10.0	–	56.2
Light cheese snack	.9 oz.	120	6.0	–	45.0
Puffed balls	1 oz.	160	10.0	–	56.2
Corn nuts	1 oz.	129	4.3	0	30.0
■Corn Puffs, fat free, Health Valley	1 oz.	100	0.0	0	0.0
■Cracker Jack	1 oz.	115	1.0	0	7.8
■Fruit Snacks, cherry, Grocer's Choice	1 oz.	99	0.0	0	0.0
■Fun Fruits, Sunkist	9 oz.	100	1.0	–	9.0
Funyuns	1 oz.	140	6.0	0	38.6

■ Contains less than 20% fat

Item	PORTION	CAL-ORIES	FAT GRAMS	CHOLES-TEROL	% OF FAT
Goldfish, tiny					
Cheddar or parmesan	1 oz.	120	4.0	5	30.0
Pretzel	1 oz.	110	3.0	0	24.5
Party mix, caracoa	1 oz.	144	8.9	37	55.6
Pork rinds, popped	1 oz.	149	8.7	37	52.6
Potato sticks	1 oz.	154	9.7	0	56.7

SOUPS

Item	PORTION	CAL-ORIES	FAT GRAMS	CHOLES-TEROL	% OF FAT
Asparagus, cream of, canned					
Prepared w/water	1 cup	85	4.1	5	43.4
Prepared w/milk	1 cup	161	7.9	22	44.2
Campbell's, prepared	1 cup	80	4.0	–	45.0
Asparagus, cream of, frozen, Kettle Ready	6 oz.	62	4.3	–	62.4
Asparagus, cream of, mix, prepared with water	1 cup	58	1.7	0	26.4
■Barley, mix, Knorr, prepared	10 oz.	120	1.8	–	13.5
■Barley Mushroom, frozen, Empire Kosher	7½ oz.	69	0.0	–	0.0
Bean w/bacon, canned					
Campbell's, prepared, regular or Special Request, less salt	1 cup	140	4.0	–	25.7
Town House, prepared	1 cup	140	4.0	–	25.7
Bean w/franks, canned, prepared w/water	1 cup	188	7.0	13	33.5

■ Contains less than 20% fat   150

Item	PORTION	CAL-ORIES	FAT GRAMS	CHOLES-TEROL	% OF FAT
Bean w/ham					
Canned, Campbell's					
Chunky, ready-to-serve	1 cup	211	6.5	–	27.7
Home Cookin', ready-to-serve	1 cup	156	3.0	–	17.3
Frozen, Kettle Ready, savory	6 oz.	113	3.6	–	28.7
Beef, canned Campbell's					
Chunky	1 cup	149	3.7	–	22.3
Prepared	1 cup	80	2.0	–	22.5
■Beef bouillon					
Cubes, dehydrated	1	6	0.1	–	15.0
Granules, Herb-Ox	1 pkg.	8	0.0	–	0.0
Beef broth, College Inn	1 cup	18	0.0	0	0.0
■Beef consommé, canned,					
Campbell's, pre-pared	1 cup	25	0.0	–	0.0
Beef noodle Canned					
Campbell's, pre-pared, home-style	1 cup	80	3.0	–	30.0
Progresso, ready-to-serve	9.5 oz.	160	4.0	–	22.5
■ Mix, Lipton, hearty, prepared	7 oz.	107	1.4	–	11.8
Beef stroganoff, canned, Campbell's, Chunky	1 cup	238	11.9	–	45.0
Beef vegetable					
■ Canned, Progresso, ready-to-serve	9.5 oz.	150	3.0	–	18.0

■ Contains less than 20% fat   151

Item	PORTION	CAL-ORIES	FAT GRAMS	CHOLES-TEROL	% OF FAT
Frozen, Kettle Ready	6 oz.	85	2.8	–	29.6
Black bean					
■ Canned, old fashioned	1 cup	87	0.4	0	4.1
■ Bean w/vegetables, fat free, Health Valley	1 cup	75	0.0	0	0.0
Frozen, Kettle Ready, w/ham	6 oz.	154	6.2	–	36.2
■ Mix, Knorr	1 cup	140	1.0	0	6.3
Borscht, Manischewitz	1 cup	80	0.0	0	0.0
Broth, chicken					
Homemade, regular, w/water	1 cup	39	1.4	0	32.3
*■ Homemade, low-fat, fat removed	1 cup	22	0.0	0	0.0
Canned					
■ Campbell's, prepared	1 cup	16	0.0	–	0.0
College Inn	1 cup	35	3.0	–	77.1
Health Valley	17 oz.	35	1.6	2	41.1
■ Health Valley, fat free	1 cup	31	0.0	0	0.0
■ Pritikin	1 cup	16	0.0	0	0.0
Swanson	7¼ oz.	18	1.0	–	50.0
■ Mix, Weight Watchers	1 pkg.	8	0.0		0.0
Cauliflower					
Frozen, Kettle Ready, cream of	6 oz.	93	6.9	–	66.8
Mix, Knorr, prepared	1 cup	100	3.0	–	27.0
Celery, cream of					
Homemade	1 cup	205	11.8	19	51.8

Item	PORTION	CAL-ORIES	FAT GRAMS	CHOLES-TEROL	% OF FAT
Canned, Campbell's, prepared	1 cup	100	7.0	–	63.0
Cheese					
Canned, Campbell's, prepared					
Cheddar	1 cup	110	6.0	–	49.1
Nacho					
Made w/milk	1 cup	180	12.0	–	60.0
Made w/water	1 cup	110	8.0	–	65.4
Frozen, Kettle Ready, cream of	6 oz.	158	12.5	–	71.2
Mix, Hain, savory, prepared	¾ cup	250	16.0	–	57.6
Chickarina, Progresso	9.5 oz.	130	5.0	20	34.6
Chicken, chunky, canned, ready-to-serve	1 cup	178	6.6	30	33.4
Campbell's, old-fashioned	1 cup	134	3.7	–	24.9
Estee, vegetable	7¼ oz.	130	7.0	30	48.5
■Chicken & corn, frozen, Empire Kosher	7½ oz.	71	1.0	–	12.7
Chicken, cream of					
Canned, Campbell's, Healthy Request, prepared w/water	8 oz.	70	2.0	10	25.7
Canned, ready-to-serve, Progresso	9½ oz.	180	11.0	–	55.0
Canned, prepared w/water, Campbell's, regular or Special Request	8 oz.	110	7.0	–	57.3

Item	PORTION	CAL-ORIES	FAT GRAMS	CHOLES-TEROL	% OF FAT
Canned, prepared w/milk	1 cup	191	11.2	27	52.8
Frozen, Kettle Ready	6 oz.	98	6.2	–	56.9
Mix, prepared w/water					
Campbell's Cup	6 oz.	90	4.0	–	40.0
Lipton Cup-A-Soup	6 oz.	84	4.4	–	47.1
Chicken gumbo					
■ Canned, ready-to-serve, Pritikin	7.4 oz.	60	1.0	5	15.0
Canned, prepared, Campbell's	1 cup	60	2.0	–	30.0
Frozen, Kettle Ready	6 oz.	93	3.5	–	38.9
■Chicken, lemon, mix, prepared w/water, Lipton Cup-A-Soup lite	6 oz.	48	0.4	4	7.5
Chicken mushroom					
Canned, prepared w/water, Campbell's creamy	1 cup	120	8.0	–	60.0
Top Ramen, chicken	1 serv.	195	8.5	–	39.2
Chicken noodle					
Canned, ready-to-serve					
Campbell's Home Cookin'	10¾ oz.	140	4.0	–	25.7
Hain, low salt	9½ oz.	110	4.0	5	32.7
Weight Watchers	10½ oz.	80	2.0	–	22.5
Canned, prepared, made w/water, Campbell's					
Regular, home-style	1 cup	70	3.0	–	38.6

Item	PORTION	CAL-ORIES	FAT GRAMS	CHOLES-TEROL	% OF FAT
Special Request	1 cup	60	2.0	15	30.0
Frozen, prepared					
■ Empire Kosher	7½ oz.	267	2.0	–	6.7
Kettle Ready	6 oz.	94	2.9	–	27.8
Mix, prepared, made w/water					
■ Knorr	1 cup	100	1.5	–	13.5
■ Lipton Cup-A-Soup					
Regular, with chicken meat	6 oz.	46	1.0	–	19.6
Hearty	6 oz.	110	1.6	–	13.1
■Chicken & pasta, mix, prepared, made w/water, Knorr	1 cup	90	1.6	–	16.0
Chicken rice					
Canned, ready-to-serve					
Campbell's					
Chunky	9½ oz.	140	4.0	–	25.7
Home Cookin'	10¾ oz.	150	6.0	–	36.0
Progresso	10½ oz.	120	4.0	25	30.0
Canned, prepared, made w/water, Campbell's, regular or Special Request	1 cup	60	3.0	–	45.0
■ Mix, made w/water, Lipton, Cup-A-Soup	6 oz.	47	0.8	–	15.3
Chicken vegetable, canned, ready-to-serve					
■ Pritikin	7¼ oz.	70	0.5	0	6.4
Progresso	9½ oz.	130	3.0	25	20.8
Chili beef					
Canned, ready-to-serve, Campbell's Chunky	11 oz.	290	7.0	–	21.7

■ Contains less than 20% fat   155

Item	PORTION	CAL-ORIES	FAT GRAMS	CHOLES-TEROL	% OF FAT
Frozen, prepared, Kettle Ready	6 oz.	161	6.5	–	36.3
Clam Chowder, Manhattan style					
*■ Homemade	1½ cups	99	0.9	18	8.1
Canned, ready-to-serve					
Campbell's Chunky	9½ oz.	150	4.0	–	24.0
■ Pritikin	7.4 oz.	70	0.5	0	6.4
Canned, prepared, Campbell's	8 oz.	70	2.0	–	25.7
Frozen, prepared					
Kettle Ready	6 oz.	69	2.6	–	33.9
■ Tabatchnick	7½ oz.	94	1.5	–	14.4
Clam chowder, New England					
Canned, ready-to-serve					
Campbell's Chunky	9½ oz.	260	15.0	–	51.9
■ Pritikin	7.4 oz.	118	0.5	0	3.8
Canned, prepared, made w/water, Campbell's	1 cup	80	3.0	–	30.0
Canned, prepared, made w/milk, Campbell's	1 cup	150	7.0	–	42.0
Frozen, prepared, Kettle Ready	6 oz.	116	6.5	–	50.4
Mix	1 pkt.	95	3.7	1	35.0
Consommé, chicken					
Canned	1 cup	39	1.4	0	32.3
■ Mix, w/gelatin	1 pkt.	78	0.1	0	1.2
Corn & broccoli chowder, frozen, prepared, Kettle Ready	6 oz.	101	5.0	–	44.5

Item	PORTION	CAL-ORIES	FAT GRAMS	CHOLES-TEROL	% OF FAT
Corn chowder, canned, ready-to-serve, Campbell's Chunky	9½ oz.	300	19.0	–	57.0
Corn chowder, prepared, made w/milk, Snow's	7½ oz.	150	6.0	–	36.0
Fish chowder, canned, prepared, made w/milk, Snow's	7½ oz.	130	6.0	–	41.5
Gazpacho					
*■ Homemade	¾ cup	35	0.2	0	5.0
Canned, ready-to-serve	1 cup	56	2.2	0	35.3
Herb, fine, mix, prepared, made w/water, Knorr	1 cup	130	6.0	–	41.5
Hot & sour, mix, oriental, prepared, Knorr	1 cup	80	3.0	–	30.0
Leek					
Dehydrated, prepared w/water	1 cup	71	2.1	3	26.6
Mix, prepared, Knorr	1 cup	110	4.0	–	32.7
Lentil					
*■ Homemade	1 cup	132	1.6	0	10.9
Canned, ready-to-serve					
■ Campbell's Home Cookin'	9½ oz.	140	1.0	–	6.4
■ Hain, regular or low sodium	9½ oz.	160	3.0	–	16.8
■ Health Valley, fat free	1 cup	75	0.0	0	0.0
Pritikin	7.4 oz.	80	0.0	0	0.0

Item	PORTION	CAL-ORIES	FAT GRAMS	CHOLES-TEROL	% OF FAT
With sausage, Progresso	9½ oz.	180	7.0	–	35.0
Mix, prepared, Hain	¾ cup	130	2.0	–	13.8
Macaroni & bean, canned, ready-to-serve, Progresso	9½ oz.	170	5.0	0	26.5
Minestrone					
■ Homemade	1 cup	113	1.7	2	13.5
Canned, ready-to-serve					
Campbell's					
Chunky	9½ oz.	160	4.0	–	22.5
■ Home Cookin', regular	10¾ oz.	140	3.0	–	19.3
Estee	7½ oz.	165	8.0	30	43.6
■ Hain, regular	9½ oz.	170	2.0	0	10.6
■ Health Valley, fat free	1 cup	85	0.0	0	0.0
■ Healthy Choice	1 cup	160	2.0	0	11.4
Pritikin	7.4 oz.	110	0.0	0	0.0
Progresso					
Beef	9½ oz.	170	5.0	–	26.5
Chicken	9½ oz.	130	3.0	20	20.8
Zesty	9½ oz.	150	8.0	10	48.0
Canned, prepared, made w/water					
Campbell's	1 cup	80	2.0	–	20.0
Town House	1 cup	80	3.0	–	30.0
Frozen, prepared					
Kettle Ready	6 oz.	104	4.4	–	38.1
■ Tabatchnick	7½ oz.	137	2.0	0	13.1
Mix, prepared					
■ Hain	¾ cup	110	1.0	–	8.2
■ Knorr	10 oz.	130	2.0	–	13.8
■ Manischewitz	6 oz.	50	0.0	–	0.0

Item	PORTION	CAL-ORIES	FAT GRAMS	CHOLES-TEROL	% OF FAT
Mushroom, cream of					
Canned, ready-to-serve					
Campbell's, Healthy Request, made w/water	8 oz.	60	2.0	5	30.0
Hain	9¼ oz.	110	4.0	15	32.7
Progresso	9.2 oz.	160	10.0	15	56.2
Weight Watchers	10½ oz.	90	2.0	–	20.0
Frozen, prepared, Kettle Ready	6 oz.	85	6.4	–	67.8
Mix, Lipton Cup-A-Soup	6 oz.	70	3.2	–	41.1
Mushroom barley, canned, ready-to-serve					
■ Hain	9½ oz.	100	2.0	10	18.0
■ Health Valley	1 cup	100	2.0	0	18.0
■ **Navy bean, canned, Pritikin**	1 cup	170	0.8	0	4.2
Onion, cream of, canned, prepared, Campbell's					
Made w/water	1 cup	100	5.0	–	45.0
Made w/water & milk	1 cup	140	7.0	–	45.0
Onion, French					
Canned, prepared, made w/water, Campbell's	1 cup	60	2.0	–	30.0
Frozen, Kettle Ready	6 oz.	42	2.2	–	47.1
Mix, prepared					
Campbell's, quality soup	1 cup	30	0.0	–	0.0
■ Knorr	1 cup	50	0.8	–	14.4
■ Lipton Cup-A-Soup	6 oz.	27	0.5	0	16.7

Item	PORTION	CAL-ORIES	FAT GRAMS	CHOLES-TEROL	% OF FAT
Oriental					
Top Ramen	1 serv.	195	8.5	0	39.2
Mix, prepared, made w/water Campbell's Cup-A-Ramen, w/vegetables					
Regular	1 cup	270	10.0	–	33.3
■ Low fat	1 cup	220	2.0	–	8.2
Lipton Cup-A-Soup lite	6 oz.	45	1.7	3	34.0
Oxtail					
Dehydrated, prepared w/water	1 cup	71	2.5	3	31.7
Mix, prepared w/water, Knorr, hearty beef	1 cup	70	2.3	–	29.6
Oyster stew, canned, prepared Campbell's					
Made w/milk	1 cup	140	9.0	–	57.9
Made w/water	1 cup	70	5.0	–	64.3
Pea soup, Tabatchnick's	7.5 oz.	174	1.9	0	9.7
Potato, canned, prepared, Campbell's, cream of					
Made w/water	1 cup	80	3.0	–	30.0
Made w/water & milk	1 cup	120	4.0	–	30.0
Schav, canned, ready-to-serve					
■ Gold's	1 cup	25	0.0	15	0.0
■ Manischewitz	1 cup	11	0.0	0	0.0
Seafood gumbo, Chauvin	8 oz.	254	11.3	120	40.0
Shrimp					
Canned, cream of, prepared, Campbell's					
Made w/water	1 cup	90	6.0	–	60.0
Made w/milk	1 cup	160	10.0	–	56.2

■ Contains less than 20% fat

Item	PORTION	CAL-ORIES	FAT GRAMS	CHOLES-TEROL	% OF FAT
■ Mix, prepared, with vegetables, Campbell's Cup-A-Ramen, low fat	1 cup	230	2.0	–	7.8
Spinach, cream of, frozen, Stouffer's	1 cup	210	15.0	–	64.3
Split pea					
Canned, ready-to-serve					
■ Anderson's	7.5 oz.	140	1.0	0	6.4
■ Campbell's, low sodium	10¾ oz.	230	4.0	–	15.6
■ Pritikin	1 cup	112	0.4	0	3.2
■ Progresso	9½ oz.	160	3.0	5	16.9
Mix, prepared w/water					
Hain	¾ cup	310	10.0	–	29.0
■ Manischewitz	6 oz.	45	0.4	–	8.0
Split pea w/ham					
Canned, prepared, made w/water, Campbell's	1 cup	160	4.0	–	22.5
Frozen, prepared, Kettle Ready	6 oz.	155	4.4	0	25.5
Steak & potato, canned, ready-to-serve, Campbell's Chunky	9½ oz.	170	4.0	–	21.2
Tomato					
Canned, ready-to-serve Campbell's					
■ Home Cookin', garden	9½ oz.	130	2.0	–	13.8
Low sodium	10½ oz.	190	6.0	–	28.4
■ Pritikin	7¼ oz.	70	0.0	0	0.0
Progresso	9½ oz.	120	3.0	0	22.5

■ Contains less than 20% fat   161

Item	PORTION	CAL-ORIES	FAT GRAMS	CHOLES-TEROL	% OF FAT
Canned, prepared, Campbell's, regular or Special Request					
Made w/milk	1 cup	150	4.0	10	24.0
Made w/water	1 cup	90	2.0	0	20.0
Frozen, Empire Kosher, Florentine	6 oz.	106	4.0	–	34.0
Mix, prepared w/water					
Hain, savory	¾ cup	220	14.0	–	57.3
Knorr, basil	1 cup	85	2.6	–	27.5
Lipton, Cup-A-Soup					
■ Regular	6 oz.	103	0.9	–	7.9
■ Lite, & herb	6 oz.	65	0.3	2	4.1
Tomato bisque, canned, prepared, Campbell	1 cup	120	3.0	–	22.5
Tomato, cream of, canned, prepared, Campbell's					
Made w/milk	1 cup	180	7.0	–	35.0
Made w/water	1 cup	110	3.0	–	24.5
■Tomato rice, canned, prepared w/water, Campbell's	1 cup	110	2.0	–	16.4
■Tomato vegetable, dehydrated, prepared w/water	1 cup	56	0.9	0	14.5
Tortellini					
Canned, ready-to-serve, Progresso					
Regular	9½ oz.	90	3.0	10	30.0
Creamy	9¼ oz.	240	16.0	35	60.0
Frozen, prepared, Kettle Ready	6 oz.	122	5.4	–	39.8
■ Mix, prepared, Knorr	1 cup	60	1.1	–	16.5
Turkey chili, frozen, Empire Kosher	7½ oz.	200	6.0	51	27.0

■ Contains less than 20% fat   162

Item	PORTION	CAL-ORIES	FAT GRAMS	CHOLES-TEROL	% OF FAT
Turkey noodle, canned, prepared w/water, Campbell's	1 cup	70	2.0	–	25.7
Turkey rice, canned, ready-to-serve, Hain, regular	9½ oz.	100	3.0	40	27.0
Turkey vegetable					
Canned, ready-to-serve					
Campbell's Chunky	9.4 oz.	150	6.0	–	36.0
Pritikin	7.4 oz.	50	0.0	5	0.0
Weight Watchers	10½ oz.	70	2.0	–	25.7
Canned, prepared, made w/water, Campbell's	1 cup	70	3.0	–	38.6
Vegetable					
Canned, ready-to-serve					
Campbell's Chunky	10¾ oz.	160	4.0	–	22.5
■ Campbell's Home Cookin'	10¾ oz.	120	2.0	–	15.0
■ Hain	9½ oz.	45	0.0	0	0.0
■ Health Valley, 14 garden, non-fat	7½ oz.	50	1.0	0	18.0
■ Pritikin	1 cup	76	0.0	0	0.0
Progresso	10½ oz.	90	2.0	5	20.0
Weight Watchers	10½ oz.	90	2.0	–	20.0
Canned, prepared, made w/water, Campbell's	1 cup	90	2.0	–	20.0
■ Frozen, Empire Kosher	7½ oz.	111	1.0	–	8.2
Mix, prepared w/water					
■ Hain, savory	¾ cup	80	1.0	–	11.2
■ Knorr	1 cup	35	0.4	–	10.3

■ Contains less than 20% fat   163

Item	PORTION	CALORIES	FAT GRAMS	CHOLESTEROL	% OF FAT
Lipton					
■ Regular, country	1 cup	80	0.7	0	7.9
■ Cup-A-Soup, harvest	6 oz.	91	1.2	0	11.9
■ Manischewitz	6 oz.	50	0.5	–	9.0
■ Vegetable barley, Health Valley, non-fat	7½ oz.	60	1.0	0	15.0
Vegetable beef					
Canned, ready-to-serve					
Campbell's					
Chunky	10¾ oz.	160	4.0	–	22.5
■ Home Cookin'	10¾ oz.	140	3.0	–	19.3
Estee, low sodium	7½ oz.	140	7.0	30	45.0
Canned, prepared w/water, Campbell's	1 cup	70	2.0	–	25.7
Vegetable, vegetarian					
Canned, ready-to-serve					
Hain					
Regular	9½ oz.	140	4.0	0	25.7
Low sodium	9½ oz.	150	5.0	0	30.0
■ Weight Watchers, chunky	10½ oz.	100	2.0	–	18.0
Vegetable broth, salt-free	1 cup	17	1.0	0	52.9
■ Vegetable broth, Swanson's	7¼ oz.	50	1.0	–	18.0
Won Ton					
Canned, prepared w/water, Campbell's	1 cup	40	1.0	–	22.5
■ Frozen, prepared, La Choy	7½ oz.	50	1.0	–	18.0

■ Contains less than 20% fat   164

SPICES & CONDIMENTS

Item	PORTION	CAL-ORIES	FAT GRAMS	CHOLES-TEROL	% OF FAT
Bacon bits, imitation, General Mills	1 tb.	37	1.4	0	34.0
■Bouquet of America	1 tsp.	4	0.0	0	0.0
■Catsup					
Del Monte	1 tb.	14	0.1	0	6.4
Heinz	1 tb.	18	0.0	0	0.0
Heinz, low-salt	1 tb.	8	0.0	0	0.0
■Chili sauce	1 tb.	16	0.0	0	0.0
Curry powder	1 tb.	20	0.9	0	40.5
■Garlic powder	1 tb.	28	0.1	0	3.2
■Horseradish, prepared	1 tb.	6	0.0	0	0.0
Mayonnaise (see Salad Dressings)					
Miso, fermented soy-bean	1 tb.	35	1.0	0	25.7
Mustard, dijon, Grey Poupon	1 tb.	18	1.0	0	50.0
Mustard, prepared					
Brown	1 tb.	14	1.0	0	64.3
Yellow, French's	1 tb.	10	1.0	0	90.0
Olives					
Black, ripe, pitted, medium	2	9	0.9	0	90.0
Green	10 gms	8	0.7	0	78.7
■Pickle					
Dill	1 med.	7	0.1	0	12.9
Sweet, whole	1 lg.	50	0.1	0	1.8
Pickle relish					
Sour, chopped	1 tb.	3	0.1	0	30.0
■ Sweet, chopped	2 tb.	42	0.2	0	4.3
■Pimiento, canned, sol-ids & liquid	2 tb.	9	0.1	0	1.0
Shake 'n' Bake					
Chicken, dry					
Original recipe	½ oz.	56	1.3	0	20.9

■ Contains less than 20% fat   165

Item	PORTION	CAL-ORIES	FAT GRAMS	CHOLES-TEROL	% OF FAT
BBQ	½ oz.	53	1.2	0	20.4
■ Fish, dry	½ oz.	55	1.0	0	16.4
■ Pork or ribs, dry, BBQ	½ oz.	54	.7	0	11.7
■Soy sauce	1 tb.	8	0.0	0	0.0
Kikkoman	1 tb.	12	0.0	0	0.0
■Tabasco sauce	1 tb.	12	0.1	0	0.0
■Teriyaki sauce Kikkoman	1 tb.	15	0.0	0	0.0
■Vinegar					
Cider	2 tb.	4	0.0	0	0.0
Distilled, white	2 tb.	4	0.0	0	0.0
■Worcestershire sauce					
French's	1 tb.	10	0.0	0	0.0
Heinz	1 tb.	15	0.0	0	0.0
Lea & Perrin's	1 tb.	10	0.0	0	0,0

VEGETABLES & LEGUMES†

Beans & Bean Products

Item	PORTION	CAL-ORIES	FAT GRAMS	CHOLES-TEROL	% OF FAT
■Baked, vegetarian, canned					
■ Campbell's	½ cup	88	0.5	0	5.0
■ S&W	½ cup	115	1.0	0	8.0
■Baked w/pork, canned					
■ Campbell's	½ cup	100	1.5	8	13.5
■ Furman's	½ cup	122	0.8	–	6.0
Hunt's	½ cup	140	1.0	1	6.4
■Baked, Barbecue B&M	½ cup	155	3.0	0	17.0
■Black, dried, cooked & drained	½ cup	114	0.0	0	0.0
■Broadbeans, mature, dried, cooked & drained	½ cup	93	0.0	0	0.0

■ Contains less than 20% fat

†There are only traces of fat in all vegetables and beans. We have listed the fat only if it is over .5 grams per serving.

Item	PORTION	CAL-ORIES	FAT GRAMS	CHOLES-TEROL	% OF FAT
■Cannellini, canned, Progresso	½ cup	80	0.0	0	0.0
■Chickpeas, dried, cooked & drained	½ cup	134	2.0	0	13.0
Fava, canned, Progresso	½ cup	90	0.0	0	0.0
■Garbanzo, canned, solids & liquid	½ cup	134	2.0	0	13.0
■Great Northern, canned, solids & liquid	½ cup	149	0.0	0	0.0
Hummus	½ cup	225	11.0	0	44.0
■Kidney, dark red, canned, w/solids & liquid	½ cup	109	0.0	0	0.0
■Lentils, dried, cooked & drained	½ cup	115	0.0	0	0.0
■Lima, baby, frozen					
Cooked & drained	½ cup	94	0.0	0	0.0
■ Uncooked, Fordhook	½ cup	85	0.0	0	0.0
■Lima, immature					
Dried, cooked & drained	½ cup	105	0.0	0	0.0
Canned, solids & liquid	½ cup	93	0.0	0	0.0
■Lima, mature, dried, cooked & drained	½ cup	108	0.0	0	0.0
■Mung, sprouted seeds, raw	½ cup	16	0.0	0	0.0
■Mung, sprouts, no seeds	½ cup	13	0.0	0	0.0
■Pinto, cooked, dried, & drained	½ cup	117	0.0	0	0.0

■ Contains less than 20% fat

Item	PORTION	CAL-ORIES	FAT GRAMS	CHOLES-TEROL	% OF FAT
■Red, dried, cooked & drained	½ cup	112	0.0	0	0.0
■Refried, canned W/bacon					
Old El Paso	½ cup	208	8.0	12	34.6
Rosarita	½ cup	132	3.0	14	20.5
W/sausage, Old El Paso	½ cup	360	16.0	–	40.0
■Refried, vegetarian, Rosarita	½ cup	120	2.0	0	15.0
■Roman, canned, Goya	½ cup	81	0.0	0	0.0
Soybeans, dried, cooked & drained	½ cup	149	7.7	0	46.5
■Split peas, cooked	½ cup	115	0.0	0	0.0
■Sprouts	½ cup	16	0.0	0	0.0
Tempeh, fermented soybean product	½ cup	165	6.4	0	34.9
Tofu, raw, firm	½ cup	183	11.0	0	54.1
■White, small, dried, cooked & drained	½ cup	127	0.6	0	4.2

Vegetables & Potatoes

Item	PORTION	CAL-ORIES	FAT GRAMS	CHOLES-TEROL	% OF FAT
■Alfalfa sprouts	½ cup	5	0.0	0	0.0
■Artichokes, fresh, cooked	1	53	0.0	0	0.0
■Artichoke hearts canned, drained	½ cup	37	0.0	0	0.0
■Asparagus					
Fresh, spears, cooked	1 each	4	0.0	0	0.0
Canned, drained	1 each	3	0.0	0	0.0
■Bamboo shoots, raw	½ cup	20	0.0	0	0.0
■Beans, green, snap					
Fresh, cooked & drained	½ cup	22	0.0	0	0.0

■ Contains less than 20% fat

Item	PORTION	CAL-ORIES	FAT GRAMS	CHOLES-TEROL	% OF FAT
Canned, solids & liquid	½ cup	18	0.0	0	0.0
Frozen, cuts, un-cooked	½ cup	20	0.0	0	0.0
Frozen, Birds Eye, cut, w/mush-rooms	5 oz.	70	2.7	8	34.7
■Beans, yellow					
Fresh, cooked & drained	½ cup	22	0.0	0	0.0
Canned, solids & liquid	½ cup	18	0.0	0	0.0
Frozen, uncooked	½ cup	20	0.0	0	0.0
■Beets					
Fresh, cooked	1	16	0.0	0	0.0
Canned, solids & liquid	½ cup	36	0.0	0	0.0
■Beets, red, pickled, canned, solids & liquid	2 tb.	18	0.0	0	0.0
■Beets, pickled, canned, solids & liquid	½ cup	74	0.0	0	0.0
■Beet Greens, (see Greens)					
■Broccoli, fresh					
Cooked	½ cup	22	0.0	0	0.0
Raw	½ cup	12	0.0	0	0.0
■Broccoli, frozen					
Plain, spears, Green Giant	½ cup (2 oz.)	12	0.0	0	0.0
In cheese sauce, Birds Eye	5 oz.	132	7.0	9	46.9
In cream sauce, Green Giant	3.3 oz.	50	1.7	2	30.6
■Brussels sprouts, fresh, cooked	½ cup	30	0.0	0	0.0

■ Contains less than 20% fat

Item	PORTION	CAL-ORIES	FAT GRAMS	CHOLES-TEROL	% OF FAT
Brussels sprouts, frozen					
With butter sauce, Green Giant	3.3 oz.	40	1.0	5	22.5
With cheese sauce, Birds Eye	4½ oz.	128	6.8	8	47.8
■Cabbage, Chinese	½ cup	5	0.0	0	0.0
■Cabbage, red					
Cooked	½ cup	16	0.0	0	0.0
Raw	½ cup	9	0.0	0	0.0
■Cabbage, white					
Cooked	½ cup	18	0.0	0	0.0
Raw	½ cup	8	0.0	0	0.0
■Carrots					
Cooked	½ cup	33	0.0	0	0.0
Raw	1	31	0.0	0	0.0
■Cauliflower					
Cooked	½ cup	15	0.0	0	0.0
Raw, florets	½ cup	19	0.0	0	0.0
■Cauliflower, frozen, w/cheese sauce, Birds Eye	4 oz.	104	5.6	9	48.5
■Celery					
Cooked, diced	½ cup	13	0.0	0	0.0
Fresh, stalk	1 each	6	0.0	0	0.0
■Chinese, raw cabbage	½ cup	34	0.0	0	0.0
Collard greens (see Greens)					
■Corn, sweet, fresh					
Yellow kernels	½ cup	90	1.0	0	10.0
White kernels	½ cup	90	1.0	0	10.0
■Corn, sweet, canned					
Cream style	½ cup	92	0.0	0	0.0
Niblets, Green Giant	½ cup	80	1.0	0	11.2
■Corn on the cob	1 med.	80	0.0	0	0.0
Corn souffle, Stouffer's	1 serv.	160	7.0	–	39.4

■ Contains less than 20% fat   170

Item	PORTION	CAL- ORIES	FAT GRAMS	CHOLES- TEROL	% OF FAT
■Cucumbers, whole, not pared	1	32	0.0	0	0.0
■Eggplant, boiled & drained	½ cup	13	0.0	0	0.0
■Endive, Belgian	½ cup	7	0.0	0	0.0
■Escarole, raw	½ cup	4	0.0	0	0.0
■Ginger root, raw	½ cup	33	0.0	0	0.0
■Greens					
Beet, fresh, boiled & drained	½ cup	19	0.0	0	0.0
Collard, cooked & drained	½ cup	12	0.0	0	0.0
Dandelion, boiled & drained	½ cup	17	0.0	0	0.9
Mustard, boiled & drained	½ cup	10	0.0	0	0.0
■ Turnip,					
Fresh, cooked	½ cup	14	0.0	0	0.0
Frozen, cooked	½ cup	25	0.0	0	0.0
■Japanese vegetables, w/seasoning, frozen, vegetable sauce, Birds Eye	½ cup	39	0.0	0	0.0
■Jerusalem artichoke, sliced, cooked	½ cup	57	0.0	0	0.0
■Kale, cooked, leaves & stems	½ cup	21	0.0	0	0.0
■Kohlrabi, thick, bulb only, cooked	½ cup	24	0.0	0	0.0
■Leeks, bulb & lower leaf, cooked	1 serv.	76	0.0	0	0.0
■Lettuce, raw					
Butterhead	½ cup	4	0.0	0	0.0
Crisphead, chopped	½ cup	4	0.0	0	0.0
Looseleaf, chopped	½ cup	5	0.0	0	0.0
■Mixed, Italian, frozen	½ cup	25	0.0	0	0.0

■ Contains less than 20% fat 171

Item	PORTION	CAL-ORIES	FAT GRAMS	CHOLES-TEROL	% OF FAT
■Mushrooms					
Fresh, raw,	1	4	0.0	0	0.0
Canned, solids & liquid	½ cup	15	0.0	0	0.0
Frozen, breaded	3 oz.	81	1.4	–	15.5
■Okra, cooked	½ cup	26	0.0	0	0.0
Onions					
Canned, French fried, Durkee	1 oz.	176	14.0	–	74.7
■ Frozen, chopped, Ore-Ida	½ cup	32	0.0	0	0.0
Onion rings	1 serv.	276	15.1	14	50.5
■Parsley, fresh, raw	½ cup	10	0.0	0	9.0
■Parsnips, boiled & diced	½ cup	63	0.0	0	2.9
■Peas & carrots, frozen, boiled & drained	½ cup	38	0.0	0	7.1
■Peas, black-eyed, cooked,	½ cup	90	0.0	0	0.0
■Peas, green, fresh, cooked	½ cup	67	0.0	0	0.0
Peas, green, canned, Le Sueur, Green Giant	½ cup	102	4.4	0	38.8
■Peas, snow, cooked	½ cup	34	0.0	0	0.0
■Peppers					
Bell, chopped	½ cup	19	0.0	0	0.0
Hot chili	½ cup	30	0.0	0	0.0
Green, chopped	½ cup	30	0.0	0	0.0
Red, chopped	½ cup	29	0.0	0	0.0
Green, chopped, sweet, raw,	½ cup	19	0.0	0	0.0
■Pimiento, canned, solids & liquid	½ cup	35	0.0	0	0.0
Potatoes, fresh					
■ Baked, w/skin	1 medium	218	0.0	0	0.0

Item	PORTION	CALORIES	FAT GRAMS	CHOLESTEROL	% OF FAT
■ Boiled	1	116	0.0	0	0.0
■ Boiled, pared, diced or sliced	½ cup	67	0.0	0	0.0
French-fried, homemade	10 pieces	158	8.3	0	40.3
Mashed, from raw, w/milk, & butter	½ cup	111	4.4	2	35.7
Potatoes, frozen					
French fried	10 pieces	111	4.4	0	25.0
Cottage Fries, Birds Eye	4 oz.	171	7.1	0	37.4
■ Birds Eye	1	37	1.3	0	3.2
■ Light, Ore-Ida	3 oz.	90	2.0	0	20.0
Skin, Ore-Ida	1 serv.	237	17.3	0	65.7
■ Hashbrowns, shred-ded, Ore-Ida	½ cup	57	0.0	–	0.0
Shoestring					
Light, Ore-Ida	3 oz.	150	6.0	–	36.0
Steak fries, Birds Eye	1	37	1.0	–	24.3
Tasti Puffs, Birds Eye	1 oz.	75	4.7	–	56.4
Tater Tots, plain, Ore-Ida	10	126	5.8	–	41.4
Tiny Taters	½ cup	151	8.9	0	53.0
Microwave, hashbrowns	3 oz.	180	10.0	0	50.0
Scalloped	½ cup	105	4.5	15	38.6
w/cheese	½ cup	162	9.3	28	51.6
Potatoes, sweet					
■ Boiled w/o skin, mashed	½ cup	172	0.0	0	0.0
Candied	1	137	3.3	0	21.7
■ Baked in skin	1	115	0.0	0	0.0
■ Yams, cooked, baked	½ cup	79	0.0	0	0.0

■ Contains less than 20% fat   173

Item	PORTION	CAL-ORIES	FAT GRAMS	CHOLES-TEROL	% OF FAT
Potatoes, au gratin					
Prepared from dry	½ cup	140	6.0	0	38.6
Betty Crocker	½ cup	140	5.0	0	32.1
Potato Buds, Betty Crocker	½ cup	130	6.0	0	41.5
Potato pancake	1	234	12.4	92	47.7
Potato Puff, frozen, cooked	4 oz.	252	12.2	0	43.6
■Pumpkin, canned	½ cup	42	0.3	0	0.0
■Radish, raw, red	1 med.	1	0.0	0	0.0
■Rutabaga, boiled, sliced	½ cup	29	0.0	0	0.0
■Sauerkraut, canned, solids & liquid	2 tb.	6	0.0	0	0.0
■Scallions, raw	½ cup	16	0.0	0	0.0
■Seaweed, kelp, raw	1 oz.	12	0.0	0	0.0
■Shallot bulbs, raw, chopped	½ cup	58	0.0	0	0.0
Spinach					
■ Raw	½ cup	6	0.0	0	0.0
Creamed	½ cup	83	4.6	3	49.9
■ Frozen, chopped, boiled & drained	½ cup	0.2	0.0	0	0.0
Spinach souffle	½ cup	109	9.2	92	74.0
■Squash					
Acorn					
Boiled, mashed	½ cup	42	0.0	0	0.0
Baked, cubed	½ cup	57	0.0	0	0.0
Butternut					
Baked, cubed	½ cup	41	0.0	0	0.0
Boiled, mashed	½ cup	49	0.0	0	0.0
Hubbard					
Cubed	½ cup	51	0.0	0	0.0
Boiled, mashed	½ cup	35	0.0	0	0.0
Summer, all types	½ cup	21	0.0	0	0.0
Zucchini, boiled	½ cup	14	0.0	0	0.0

■ Contains less than 20% fat

Item	PORTION	CAL-ORIES	FAT GRAMS	CHOLES-TEROL	% OF FAT
■Succotash, frozen, boiled & drained	½ cup	79	0.0	0	0.0
■Swiss chard					
Raw	½ cup	3	0.0	0	0.0
Cooked	½ cup	17	0.0	0	0.0
■Tomatoes					
Raw	1	26	0.0	0	0.0
Canned, ripe, solids & liquid	½ cup	24	0.0	0	0.0
Stewed	½ cup	30	0.0	0	0.0
■Tomato paste, canned	½ cup	110	1.1	0	9.0
■Tomato puree, canned, regular	½ cup	49	0.0	0	0.0
Turnip					
Raw	½ cup	18	0.0	0	0.0
Boiled, cubed	½ cup	14	0.1	0	0.0
■Water chestnut					
Canned, sliced, solids & liquid	½ cup	35	0.0	0	0.0
Chinese, raw	1	10	0.0	0	0.0
■Watercress, raw, chopped	½ cup	2	0.0	0	0.0

PREPARED FOODS

Item	PORTION	CAL-ORIES	FAT GRAMS	CHOLES-TEROL	% OF FAT
Beans & franks, canned, solids & liquid	1 cup	365	16.9	15	41.7
Bean & frankfurter dinner, frozen					
Banquet	10 oz.	520	25.0	35	43.3
Swanson 3-compartment	10½ oz	440	19.0	–	38.9
■Beef Americana, Light Balance	8¼ oz.	190	3.0	14	14.2

■ Contains less than 20% fat   175

Item	PORTION	CAL-ORIES	FAT GRAMS	CHOLES-TEROL	% OF FAT
■Beef and pasta Bordeaux, Light Balance	8¼ oz.	181	0.9	25	4.5
Beef, creamed, chipped, cooked	1 cup	377	25.2	98	60.2
Beef, creamed, chipped, frozen, Swanson	11 oz.	460	32.0	–	62.6
Beef, oriental					
Hormel Top Shelf	10.3 oz.	290	10.0	–	31.0
Hunt's Entree Maker	7.6 oz.	271	12.0	–	39.8
Beef, pepper oriental, canned, La Choy	¾ cup	90	2.0	–	20.0
Beef stew, homemade w/vegetables,	1 serv.	186	7.5	40	36.3
Beef stew, canned					
w/vegetables	1 cup	194	7.3	34	33.9
Dinty Moore	3.5 oz.	80	3.8	–	42.7
Estee, dietetic	7½ oz.	210	11.0	30	47.1
Beef, stir-fried w/vegetables, homemade	8 oz.	200	7.7	39	34.6
Beef, stroganoff, Kraft, w/noodles, microwaveble meal	9 oz.	310	12.0	–	34.8
Burrito, beef	1	262	10.4	32	35.7
Cheese fondue, homemade	1 cup	697	47.8	589	61.7
Chicken a la king					
Homemade	1 cup	468	34.3	186	66.0
Canned, Swanson	5¼ oz.	190	12.0	–	56.8
Chicken Acapulco, Top Shelf	10 oz.	410	16.0	–	35.1

■ Contains less than 20% fat

176

Item	PORTION	CAL-ORIES	FAT GRAMS	CHOLES-TEROL	% OF FAT
Chicken and noodles, homemade	1 cup	367	18.2	96	44.6
Chicken cacciatore	1 serv.	287	18.6	63	58.3
■Chicken cacciatore w/pasta Light Balance	1 serv.	206	0.9	25	3.9
Chicken fettuccini, Kraft, micro-wave entree	9 oz.	270	13.0	–	43.4
Chicken fried steak w/gravy	1 serv.	324	20.0	84	55.5
Chicken, stir-fried and almonds, homemade	8 oz.	243	9.1	68	33.7
■Chicken, sweet and sour, w/rice, Kraft	10 oz.	250	1.0	–	3.6
■Chili, chunky turkey	1 serv.	216	3.8	20	15.8
Chili w/beans					
Canned, solids & liquid	1 cup	286	14.0	43	44.0
Health Valley	8 oz.	208	4.8	0	208
Healthy Choice	7.5 oz.	200	5.0	–	22.5
Hormel, micro-wave, hot	7.4 oz.	250	11.0	–	39.6
Just Rite, hot	8 oz.	390	20.0	66	46.1
Lunch Bucket, mi-crowave	8½ oz.	340	16.0	45	42.3
Chili w/o beans, canned					
Gebhardt	7½ oz.	410	32.0	–	70.2
Hormel	7½ oz.	270	28.0	–	93.3
Just Rite	8 oz.	360	22.0	82	55.0
Old El Paso	1 cup	162	7.0	47	38.9
Chili, mix, prepared, Manwich Chili Fixins	8 oz.	290	14.0	65	43.4

■ Contains less than 20% fat

Item	PORTION	CAL-ORIES	FAT GRAMS	CHOLES-TEROL	% OF FAT
Chili, vegetarian, no salt, Health Valley	1 cup	358	19.9	0	50.0
■ w/Black Beans, fat-free, Health Valley	5 oz.	140	0.0	0	0.0
Chop suey w/meat, canned	1 cup	155	8.0	30	46.4
Chow mein, beef, no noodles	1 serv.	295	18.9	59	57.7
Chow mein, chicken, no noodles	1 serv.	275	15.6	64	51.0
Coq au vin, ¼ chicken, 1 cup vegetables	1 serv.	663	28.1	260	38.1
Corned beef hash	2 oz.	293	17.3	88	53.0
■Dinosaurs, Chef Boyardee	7.5 oz.	180	1.0	–	5.0
Egg foo yung dinner, canned, La Choy, prepared	1 patty + ¼ cup sauce	164	7.0	–	38.4
Egg roll	1	129	5.9	64	41.2
Frozen, La Choy					
Chicken	.5 oz.	30	1.0	–	30.0
Lobster	3 oz.	180	5.0	–	25.0
Shrimp	.5 oz.	27	0.7	–	23.3
Eggplant parmigiana, FSC	2 oz.	336	23.8	85	63.7
Enchilada, cheese	1	319	18.8	44	53.0
Falafel ball or patty	1	57	3.0	0	47.4
Fettucini Alfredo, homemade	1 cup	403	24.8	102	55.4
Hamburger Helper, prepared					
Beef noodle	⅓ of pkg.	325	15.0	–	42.2
Cheeseburger macaroni	⅓ of pkg.	350	16.0	–	41.1
Hamburger hash	⅓ of pkg.	320	15.0	–	42.2

■ Contains less than 20% fat

Item	PORTION	CAL-ORIES	FAT GRAMS	CHOLES-TEROL	% OF FAT
Meatloaf	⅓ of pkg.	360	22.0	–	55.0
Hash, turkey	1 serv.	339	8.5	58	22.6
Lasagna					
Homemade	6 oz.	304	11.9	58	35.2
w/sauce	8 oz.	347	12.5	50	32.4
Hormel, microcup	3.5 oz.	122	7.1	–	52.3
■Lasagna, frozen w/meat sauce, Healthy Choice	9 oz.	250	4.0	20	14.4
Lasagna, vegetarian, cheese	6 oz.	313	14.4	45	41.4
■Macaroni & beef, Lunch Bucket	8½ oz.	250	4.0	–	14.4
Macaroni and cheese					
Baked, homemade	1 cup	506	27.2	83	48.4
Deluxe, prepared, Kraft	1 cup	340	10.9	26	28.8
Eating Right, Kraft	9 oz.	270	8.0	15	26.7
Elbow, Franco-American	1 cup	170	6.0	–	31.8
Frozen, Campbell's	9 oz.	276	12.2	2	39.8
Prepared, Kraft	1 cup	402	18.6	6	41.6
■Manicotti	1 cup	227	5.0	17	19.8
Meatloaf					
Prepared w/ground beef	1 serv.	258	15.6	124	54.4
■ Prepared w/ground turkey	1 serv.	175	3.0	40	15.4
Mushroom stroganoff, Light Balance	8¼ oz.	190	6.0	–	28.4
■Pasta w/garden vegetables, Light Balance	8 ¼ oz.	170	1.0	2	5.3
Pâté de foie gras, canned	1 cup	960	90.8	910	85.1
Pepper Steak	3 oz.	256	14.9	70	52.4

■ Contains less than 20% fat

Item	PORTION	CAL-ORIES	FAT GRAMS	CHOLES-TEROL	% OF FAT
Pizza, cheese, ⅛ of 12″ pie	1 slice	109	2.5	7	20.6
Pizza, French bread, cheese	1 serv.	340	13.0	–	34.4
■ Healthy Choice	5.6 oz.	300	3.0	–	9.0
Pot pie, beef, home-made, baked	1 serv.	556	32.8	47	53.1
■Ravioli					
Canned	1 cup	240	7.3	20	20.0
Beef, Chef Boyardee	7.5 oz.	190	4.0	–	18.9
Cheese, Chef Boyardee	7.5 oz.	200	3.0	–	13.5
Hormel Microcup	7½ oz.	250	11.0	–	39.6
■Rice, fried, Chinese, no meat, home-made	1 cup	206	3.3	45	14.4
Salisbury steak, Hormel Top Shelf	10 oz.	340	19.0	–	50.3
Spaghetti and meat-balls, Chef Boyardee	4.5 oz.	119	4.0	–	30.2
■Spaghetti, homemade					
w/meat sauce	1 cup	218	4.7	34	19.4
w/tomato sauce, cheese	1 cup	260	8.7	7	30.1
■Spaghetti, canned					
w/plain sauce, Ragu	1 cup	266	3.6	–	12.2
w/tomato sauce, cheese	1 cup	190	1.5	7	7.1
■Spaghetti, frozen, Healthy Choice	7.5 oz.	150	3.0	–	18.0
■SpaghettiOs, Franco-American	7.37 oz.	160	2.0	–	11.2

Item	PORTION	CALORIES	FAT GRAMS	CHOLESTEROL	% OF FAT
Stroganoff, beef, w/o noodles	1 serv.	332	23.9	78	64.8
Stroganoff, mushroom, Light Balance	1 serv.	183	4.4	11	21.6
Taco	1 small	369	20.6	56	50.2
*■Tamale pie	1 serv.	352	4.8	21	12.3
Tamale, canned	3 oz.	119	6.0	–	45.4
Tortellini, cheese, w/shrimp & seafood, Hormel Top Shelf	10 oz.	280	8.0	–	25.7
Tuna Helper, prepared					
Au gratin	⅕ of pkg.	280	11.0	–	35.3
Cheesy noodles	⅕ of pkg.	250	9.0	–	32.4
Tetrazzini	⅕ of pkg.	240	8.0	–	30.0
Welsh Rarebit, frozen, Stouffer's	4 oz.	288	23.8	–	74.4

DINING OUT

THE DINER'S DILEMMA QUIZ

Dining out need not be fattening or hazardous to your health. Try taking your good habits and this book to the restaurant with you.

Each of us is more in control of our health than we realize. Take this quiz to determine your health I.Q.:

T F You are someone who eats everything you feel like eating—someone who "lives to eat."

T F You think of yourself as a "meat and potatoes" person, and include animal protein at every meal.

T F You avoid whole grains, salads, and fresh vegetables whenever possible.

T F You think of "breadandbutter" as one word.

T F You never miss a chance to have a rich dessert, and feel that no meal is complete without one.

T F You seldom read the labels on the foods you buy, so your pantry shelves are filled with processed and refined foods.

T F You go to fast food places at least once a week, eating mostly hamburgers, hot dogs, french fries, and pizzas.

T F You feel a low-fat, low-cholesterol diet just means avoiding eggs and red meat.

T F Whenever you get the urge to exercise, you relax and wait until the feeling passes.

T F You count on the fact that if you ever develop a health problem, a drug or some "medical miracle" will save you.

If you answered true to some or all of these questions, it's time to make some changes when eating out.

Don't be discouraged if you're not perfect. A healthy lifestyle isn't built overnight.

Item	PORTION	CALORIES	FAT GRAMS	CHOLESTEROL	% OF FAT
Chinese					
Beef					
w/broccoli	4 oz. beef	315	19.0	65	54.3
w/oyster sauce	3 oz. beef	265	15.0	49	50.9
Szechuan style, w/red hot chiles, carrot strips and bamboo shoots	4 oz. beef	345	17.0	65	44.3
Buns, Chinese steamed	1 each	190	8.0	0	37.9
Chicken					
Skinned and boneless w/black bean sauce and peppers	4 oz. chicken	480	27.0	85	50.6
w/cashew nuts or walnuts	4 oz. chicken	575	35.0	85	54.8
Kung Pao	3½ oz. chicken	566	50.0	130	79.5
Moo Goo Gai Pan	1 cup	304	17.2	66	57.0
Cookie					
Almond	1 each	118	6.9	12	52.6
■ Fortune	1 each	23	0.2	–	7.8
Duck, Peking	1 serv.	351	24.1	71	61.8
Dumplings, fried (pot stickers)					
Chicken filled	1 each	57	2.8	11	44.2
Shrimp and pork filled	1 each	53	1.8	9	30.6
Egg Foo Yung	⅓ of 6-egg dish	180	12.0	330	60.0
Egg Roll	1 each	153	10.5	64	59.0
Fish					
■ Snapper, steamed	3 oz.	85	1.1	31	11.6
Sweet and sour	1 serv.	274	15.0	58	49.1
Fried bananas w/sweet sauce	1 serv.	304	17.2	66	50.0

Item	PORTION	CAL-ORIES	FAT GRAMS	CHOLES-TEROL	% OF FAT
Noodles chow mein, canned	½ cup	119	6.9	0	52.2
Pork					
Barbecued	1 serv.	201	7.8	51	35.0
Sweet and sour	4 oz. meat	470	25.0	145	47.9
Twice cooked	4 oz. meat	300	20.0	75	60.0
Rice					
Fried, w/pork	1 cup	330	15.0	230	40.9
■ Steamed	1 cup	220	2.0	0	9.0
Shellfish					
Crab w/black bean sauce	12–16 oz. crab in shell	325	24	110	66.5
Hot and sour shrimp	4 oz.	235	12.0	130	46.0
Lobster Cantonese	6 oz. in shell	295	17.0	180	51.9
Shrimp w/snow peas	4 oz. shrimp	245	12.0	130	44.1
Soup					
Hot and sour w/tofu	1 cup	198	10.0	0	45.4
Wonton	1 cup	107	4.1	69	34.5
Spareribs					
Barbecued	1 serv.	252	17.1	69	61.9
w/black bean sauce	8 oz. ribs	325	25.0	65	69.2
Vegetables					
■ Chinese, steamed	1 cup	68	0.3	0	4.0
Lo Mein	1 cup	185	7.2	11	34.0
Stir-fried (cloud ears, broccoli, carrots and water chestnuts)	1 cup	135	7.5	0	50.0
Stir-fried eggplant, w/sesame sauce	6 oz. eggplant	205	15.0	0	65.8

■ Contains less than 20% fat

Item	PORTION	CAL-ORIES	FAT GRAMS	CHOLES-TEROL	% OF FAT
Coffee Shop (see Denny's, p. 69)					
Chinese chicken salad	1 cup	203	10.9	22	48.0
Sandwiches					
Club	1	590	20.8	52	31.3
w/mayonnaise					
Egg salad	1	279	12.5	228	38.0
Grilled cheese	1	680	44.0	77	58.0
w/bacon					
Ham	1	281	9.8	29	29.0
w/mayonnaise					
Reuben	1	531	33.3	77	56.0
Tuna melt	1	900	49.0	71	50.0
Tuna salad	1	278	14.2	10	45.0
■ Turkey breast	1	285	5.2	15	15.5
w/mustard					
Turkey	1	402	18.4	17	40.1
w/mayonnaise					
Delicatessen					
■Applesauce	¼ cup	50	0.5	0	9.0
■Bagel, 3″ Plain	1 (1.9 oz.)	162	1.0	0	5.5
■Bialy	1	80	0.0	0	0.0
Blintzes, Plain					
Cottage cheese	1	130	4.5	75	31.1
Pot cheese	1	126	3.5	65	25.0
Ricotta cheese	1	150	7.5	85	45.0
Topping					
■ Dark cherry sauce	¼ cup	90	0.0	0	0.0
Sour cream	2 tb.	50	5.0	16	90.0
Bread					
Challah	1-oz. slice	120	3.0	35	22.5
■ Pumpernickel	1-oz. slice	80	1.0	0	11.2
■ Rye	1.1-oz. slice	80	1.0	0	11.2
Brisket of beef, boiled	4 oz.	260	14.0	100	48.5

■ Contains less than 20% fat

Item	PORTION	CAL-ORIES	FAT GRAMS	CHOLES-TEROL	% OF FAT
Chicken in pot w/vegetables	1 serv.	611	29.7	201	44.8
Chicken liver					
Chopped	⅓ cup	175	11.0	540	58.0
Sauteed (2 oz. liver)	1 serv.	130	8.0	250	55.4
Coleslaw	1 cup	173	16.8	10	87.4
Corned beef hash	1 cup	374	24.4	80	59.6
Cream cheese	1 oz.	106	10.7	31	90.8
Danish pastry					
Apple	3 oz.	240	8.0	–	30.0
Cheese	4.5 oz.	380	22.0	–	52.1
■Gefilte fish in natural broth	2-oz. piece	46	0.8	–	15.6
Herring					
Pickled	3 oz.	190	13.0	85	61.5
w/sour cream	1 serv.	133	10.1	40	67.7
Knish, potato	1	73	3.2	–	39.2
Knockwurst	4 oz.	410	37.8	72	71.2
*■Lox (smoked salmon)	3 oz.	100	3.7	20	19.0
Potato pancake	2 oz.	175	30.0	70	95.0
■Rice pudding w/raisins	½ cup	190	4.2	35	18.9
Rugelach, maple nut	1	98	6.0	45	55.1
Salad					
Macaroni	½ cup	349	23.4	136	60.3
Potato	½ cup	237	17.3	47	65.7
Sandwiches					
* Corned beef on rye	4 oz. meat	582	21.3	110	45.0
Pastrami (lean) on rye	4 oz. meat	396	19.5	105	44.0
Salami	4 oz. meat	460	40.0	120	78.0
■ Turkey breast	4 oz. meat	310	3.6	78	10.4
Soup					
Chicken w/matzo balls	1 cup	271	14.8	174	49.2

Item	PORTION	CAL-ORIES	FAT GRAMS	CHOLES-TEROL	% OF FAT
■ Chicken w/rice	1 cup	165	3.5	31	19.1
■ Mushroom barley	1 cup	139	1.0	0	6.5
■ Split pea	1 cup	158	1.0	0	5.7
■ Salmon	4 oz.	208	12.4	55	52.0
Sturgeon, smoked	4 oz.	196	5.0	–	22.9
■Whitefish, smoked	4 oz.	122	1.1	–	8.1
French					
Bananas flambé	1 banana	465	20.0	60	38.7
Beef Provençal	4 oz. beef	265	15.0	65	50.9
Bouillabaisse (made w/fish fillets, shrimp, crab or lobster and clams or oysters)	4 oz. fish	120	3.0	80	22.5
Caviar	1 tsp.	26	1.5	47	51.0
Cherries Jubilee	½ cup	190	7.0	30	33.2
■Chicken breast, poached, w/tomato coulis	1 each	161	3.3	73	18.4
Chicken cordon bleu	1 each	310	12.0	150	34.8
Coquilles St. Jacques	4 oz. scallops	400	26.0	130	58.4
Crepes					
Plain	1	50	3.0	60	54.0
Filled with creamed chicken	1	185	10.0	95	48.6
Crepes Suzette	1	310	17.0	100	49.3
Duck à l'orange	1 serv. (¼ of 4½–5 lb. duck)	1,010	68.0	170	60.6
Escargots	4	150	15.0	8	90.0
Lamb, rack, lean	3 oz.	184	8.3	81	40.6
■Meringue shells w/fruit	1	114	0.3	0	2.4

■ Contains less than 20% fat   188

Item	PORTION	CALORIES	FAT GRAMS	CHOLESTEROL	% OF FAT
Mousse, chocolate, homemade	1 cup	434	25.0	288	51.8
Paté de foi gras	1 oz.	131	12.4	43	84.7
Quiche Lorraine	⅙ of 9" pie	520	35.0	250	60.6
Ratatouille, vegetable medley	1 serv.	98	5.8	0	53.3
Salmon, poached	3 oz.	121	5.4	47	40.1
■Sorbet, orange	?	110	0.1	0	1.0
Souffle					
Cheese	1 serv.	380	25.0	310	59.2
Lemon, chilled, w/whipped cream	½ cup	290	15.0	120	46.5
Soup, onion, au gratin	1 serv.	284	15.6	27	49.4
Truffle, chocolate	1	135	11.6	17	77.3
Italian					
Biscuit Tortoni	1	235	23.0	53	88.1
Bread					
Garlic	1 slice	111	4.3	1	34.9
■ Italian	.8-oz. slice	175	1.0	–	6.7
Stick, sesame	1	50	2.0	0	36.0
Calamari, fried	3 oz.	175	7.5	201	39.0
Cannelloni	1 serv.	420	29.0	185	60.2
Cappuccino	4 fl. oz.	40	1.5	10	33.7
Cheese, parmesan, grated	1 tb.	23	1.5	4	58.7
Eggplant Parmesan	1 serv.	356	24.0	31	60.6
Fettuccini Alfredo	1 serv. (2 oz. dry noodles)	650	44.0	70	60.9
Gnocci					
Potato	6	550	31.0	150	50.7
Ricotta (Malfatti)	4	460	20.0	150	39.1
■Ice, Italian	3 fl. oz.	86	0.0	0	0.0

■ Contains less than 20% fat   189

Item	PORTION	CAL-ORIES	FAT GRAMS	CHOLES-TEROL	% OF FAT
Lasagna w/beef & cheese	1 serv.	400	19.8	81	45.0
Linguini w/clam sauce					
■ Red	1 serv.	292	3.9	10	12.0
White	1 serv.	346	12.9	15	33.6
Manicotti	1 serv.	238	11.8	61	44.2
Mozzarella, fried, w/marinara sauce	1 serv.	591	45.2	45	68.8
Mussels Marinara	10 oz. mussels	210	8.0	25	34.3
■Polenta	1 cup	85	0.8	0	8.4
Ravioli, w/meat	1	49	3.0	19	56.0
Salads					
■ Arugula & Belgian endive	1 cup	14	0.0	0	0.0
Caesar	1 cup	292	29.7	2	91.5
House, w/cheese and salami	1 serv.	607	53.4	45	79.2
Mozzarella and to-mato	1 serv.	185	12.7	44	61.8
■ Tomato and onion	1 serv.	53	0.5	0	8.5
Sausage, Italian	2 oz.	216	17.2	52	80.0
Soup					
Minestrone	10 oz. (1¼ cups)	180	5.0	0	25.0
Tortellini w/escarole, in broth	1 serv.	300	8.0	38	24.0
Spaghetti					
Al pesto	2 cups cooked	740	34.0	6	41.3
Carbonara	4 oz. dry	1090	65.0	505	53.7
w/marinara sauce	1 serv.	383	10.1	0	22.4
Primavera	1 serv.	180	7.0	30	35.0
■ w/tomato and basil	1 serv.	226	1.4	0	5.5
Tiramisu	1 serv.	240	16.0	170	60.0

■ Contains less than 20% fat   190

Item	PORTION	CAL-ORIES	FAT GRAMS	CHOLES-TEROL	% OF FAT
Veal					
Parmigiana	4 oz. veal	500	30.0	210	54.0
w/peppers	1 serv.	380	29.0	100	68.7
Scaloppine marsala	1 serv.	450	21.0	185	42.0
■ Shank, baked, w/risotto	1 serv.	490	10.0	130	18.4
Vegetables					
Broccoli, sauteed w/garlic and oil	1 serv.	75	5.0	0	60.0
Escarole, braised	1 serv.	60	4.0	10	60.0
■ Peppers, roasted	½ cup	25	0.0	0	0.0
Zabaglione	1 serv.	77	3.5	145	41.0
Mexican					
Bananas Managua w/Mexican cream	1 serv. (½ banana)	255	15.0	45	52.9
Beans, refried	½ cup	100	6.0	0	54.0
Burrito, no cheese					
■ Bean	1 each	145	3.0	–	18.6
■ Lentil	1 each	239	4.0	0	15.1
Chicken breast, boneless, w/mole sauce	1 breast	250	10.0	80	36.0
Chili con carne	1 cup	328	13.8	54	37.9
Chimichanga	1 each	242	14.2	–	52.8
Coffee, Mexican mocha	6 oz.	390	14.0	10	32.3
Empanada, turkey or chicken	1 (6½"–7" wide)	550	30.0	123	49.1
Enchilada					
Beef	1 each	530	28.0	80	47.5
Chicken	1 serv.	510	17.0	–	30.0
Fajita					
Beef	1	306	15.0	32	44.1
Beef and vegetable	1	240	7.5	28	28.1
Chicken	1	235	11.5	39	44.0

■ Contains less than 20% fat　　191

Item	PORTION	CALORIES	FAT GRAMS	CHOLESTEROL	% OF FAT
Flan	½ cup	95	3.2	90	30.3
Frijoles–zucchini tortilla pie	1	410	19.0	80	41.7
Guacamole dip	1 tb.	34	3.1	2	82.0
Huevos Rancheros	2 eggs	465	15.0	565	29.0
Menudo	1 serv.	278	8.2	192	25.9
Nachos, vegetable	1	30	2.0	2	60.0
Quesadillas, grilled	1	250	16.0	24	57.6
Salsa	1 tb.	12	1.0	0	75.0
■Sangria	¾ cup	210	0.0	0	0.0
Sopai pillas (deep-fried dough w/sugar)	1	88	6.0	0	61.0
Soup					
Black bean	1 cup	240	6.0	5	22.5
Gazpacho	1 cup	56	2.2	0	35.4
Nacho beef and cheese	1 cup	400	25.0	80	56.2
Taco, Beef	1	230	15.0	45	58.7
■Tortilla, soft, w/salsa	1 serv.	81	1.2	0	13.3
Tortilla chips w/salsa	1 serv.	149	7.5	0	45.3
Tostados, beef, w/guacamole and salsa	1	480	27.0	50	50.6
Middle Eastern					
Falafel	1 oz.	115	6.0	–	47.0
Feta cheese	1 oz.	75	4.0	25	48.0
■Gyro Sandwich	1 (3 oz. meat)	460	10.0	60	19.6
■Pita bread					
Wheat	2 oz. pc.	150	2.0	0	12.0
White	2 oz. pc.	158	1.0	0	5.7
Shish Kabobs, Lamb	1 (4 oz. meat)	180	13.0	70	65.0

■ Contains less than 20% fat

Item	PORTION	CAL-ORIES	FAT GRAMS	CHOLES-TEROL	% OF FAT
Seafood					
Butter					
Regular	1 pat	36	4.1	11	100.0
Clarified	1 tb.	110	12.0	30	98.2
Clams					
Casino	6	245	24.8	85	91.1
Fried	4 oz.	320	18.0	130	50.6
■ Raw	6 each	90	1.0	40	10.0
■ Steamers, no butter	1 doz.	180	1.0	80	5.0
Crab					
■ Alaskan king crab claws, steamed	3½ oz.	96	1.5	53	14.0
Deviled	1 serv.	270	19.0	130	63.3
Soft shell, sauteed	1	159	9.5	65	53.8
Flounder or sole fillets					
Broiled	4 oz.	170	8.0	70	42.3
Fried	4 oz.	375	25.0	150	60.0
Lobster					
Newburg	2 oz. lobster	400	30.0	260	67.5
■ Tail, broiled, no butter	8-oz. tail	110	1.0	100	12.2
Thermidor	1 serv.	150	6.0	50	36.0
■ Whole, boiled	1-lb. lobster	100	2.0	90	18.0
Mussels marinara	9-oz. serv.	210	8.0	26	34.3
Oysters					
Fried	4 oz.	300	18.0	120	54.0
Raw	6 each	80	3.0	60	33.7
Scalloped	4 oz.	280	16.0	60	51.4
Oyster stew	8 oz.	410	25.0	110	54.9
Potato					
■ Baked, plain, w/skin	1	218	0.0	0	0.0
French fries	2 oz.	156	7.5	–	43.3
Redfish, blackened	4 oz.	133	2.4	61	16.0
Rice pilaf	½ cup	130	7.0	0	39.0

■ Contains less than 20% fat

Item	PORTION	CALORIES	FAT GRAMS	CHOLESTEROL	% OF FAT
■Rice, plain, white	½ cup	135	0.7	0	4.7
Salmon, poached, w/lemon Sauce	6 oz.	280	15.0	70	48.2
■ Seafood cocktail	1 tb.	12	0.0	0	0.0
Tartar	1 tb.	70	7.0	4	90.0
■Scallops, grilled	4 oz.	81	1.2	30	13.0
Shrimp					
■ Batter fried	4 oz.	170	3.0	200	15.9
■ Boiled	⅓ lb.	100	1.0	170	9.0
Creole	1 serv.	390	15.0	90	34.6
French fried	7 med.	200	10.0	168	45.0
Soup, chowder					
Clam					
Manhattan	8 oz.	160	4.0	35	22.5
New England	8 oz.	230	7.0	50	27.4
Fish	8 oz.	330	10.0	60	27.3
Shrimp gumbo	8 oz.	155	3.9	40	23.0
Sour cream	1 tb.	25	2.5	8	90.0
■Surimi (imitation crab and shrimp)	3 oz.	84	1.0	25	10.0
Trout, pan fried, rainbow	¼ of 8-oz. fish	400	20.0	180	45.0

Thai

Item	PORTION	CALORIES	FAT GRAMS	CHOLESTEROL	% OF FAT
Cabbage, spinach and tofu in peanut sauce over rice noodles	1 serv.	545	28.0	0	46.2
Chicken w/basil and coconut milk	4½ oz. chicken	320	17.0	65	47.8
Chicken wings w/garlic sauce	4 pieces (2 whole wings)	410	20.0	160	43.9

■ Contains less than 20% fat   194

Item	PORTION	CAL-ORIES	FAT GRAMS	CHOLES-TEROL	% OF FAT
Noodles, (Mee Krab) Crunchy, w/chicken, pork and shrimp	1 serv.	550	15.0	160	24.5
Soft fried, w/pork, shrimp and vegetables	1 serv.	560	30.0	205	48.2
Shark or swordfish w/coconut sauce	4 oz. cooked fish	305	19.0	70	56.1
Shrimp salad w/coconut and ginger	4 oz.	247	14.0	140	51.0

By the year 2000, 2 out of 3 Americans could be illiterate.

It's true.

Today, 75 million adults...about one American in three, can't read adequately. And by the year 2000, U.S. News & World Report envisions an America with a literacy rate of only 30%.

Before that America comes to be, you can stop it...by joining the fight against illiteracy today.

Call the Coalition for Literacy at toll-free **1-800-228-8813** and volunteer.

Volunteer Against Illiteracy. The only degree you need is a degree of caring.